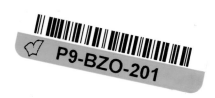

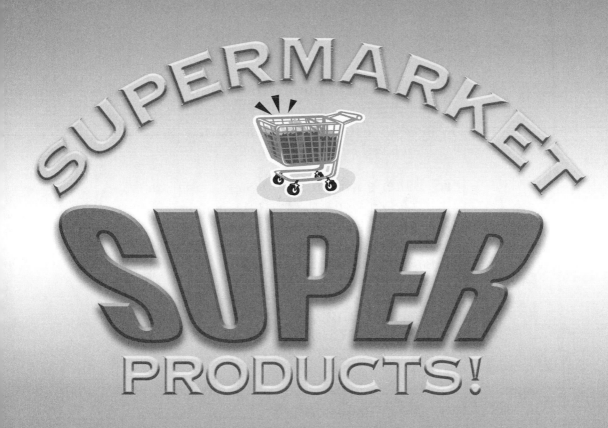

# SUPERMARKET SUPER PRODUCTS!

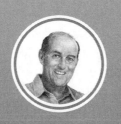

www.jerrybaker.com

# SUPERMARKET SUPER PRODUCTS!

## 2,568 SUPER SOLUTIONS, TERRIFIC TIPS & REMARKABLE RECIPES FOR GREAT HEALTH, A HAPPY HOME, AND A BEAUTIFUL GARDEN

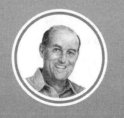

## BY JERRY BAKER

Published by American Master Products, Inc.

# Copyright © 2003 by Jerry Baker

**Published by American Master Products, Inc. / Jerry Baker**
**Executive Editor:** Kim Adam Casior
**Managing Editor:** Cheryl Winters Tetreau
**Writer:** Vicki Webster
**Copy Editor:** Barbara McIntosh Webb
**Interior Design and Layout:** Nancy Biltcliff
**Cover Design:** Kitty Pierce Mace
**Indexer:** Nan Badgett
Some images in this book were sourced from Clipart.com.

**Publisher's Cataloging-in-Publication**

Baker, Jerry.
    Supermarket super products! : 2,568 super solutions, terrific tips
& remarkable recipes for great health, a happy home, and a beautiful
garden / [Jerry Baker].
    p. cm. – (A Jerry Baker living well book)
    Includes index.

    1. Home economics. 2. Health 3. Gardening. I. Title.

TX145.B29 2003         640'.41
           QBI03-200331

Printed in the United States of America
6 8 10 9 7 5 hardcover

# SUPER IS AS SUPER DOES!

*I've got a little teaser for you: What do
the following 5 things have in common?*

1. A skin-softening, nourishing facial masque
2. No-muss, no-fuss silver polish
3. Gleefully gory, Halloween monster makeup
4. Guaranteed frost protection for your car's windshield
5. A potent pest killer that's so safe, you can eat it!

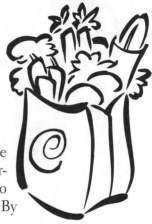

***Are you ready for the answer?*** It's easy: You can make
every one of these wonders with items found at your local supermarket. And you probably buy them almost every week! So how do
you tap into the magic power of that stuff in your shopping cart? By
using my fast, fun, and easy directions that follow.

This book is jam-packed with thousands of tips, tricks, and tonics for putting
these super-powered super products to work in your home, garage, and yard, and even
on your family. I'll give you the lowdown on:

🍎 Old-time and new-fangled health and beauty treatments that
beat commercial versions, hands down.

◆ Simple, nontoxic cleaners, polishers, and stain removers that'll
spruce up your whole house—and everything in it.

▦ Treats and toys that are *guaranteed* to delight the daylights out
of your kids, grandkids, and pets.

▼ Super secrets that'll make workshop projects a breeze, and
keep the old jalopy looking as good as the day you brought it home
(well, almost as good).

● Excellent elixirs that'll help make your outdoor green scene a
regular Garden of Eden.

***But wait—there's even more!*** You'll also discover hundreds of ways to turn
potential trash into handy household helpers, great garden gadgets, or pet- and people-
pleasing playthings. They're fast and easy, too!

***So what are we waiting for? Let the fun begin!***

# CONTENTS

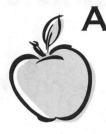

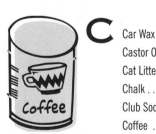

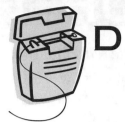

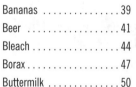
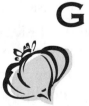
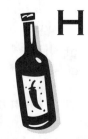
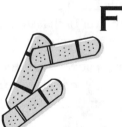

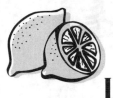

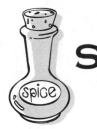

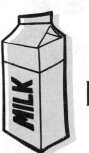

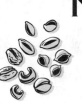

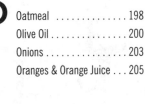

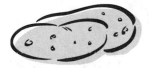

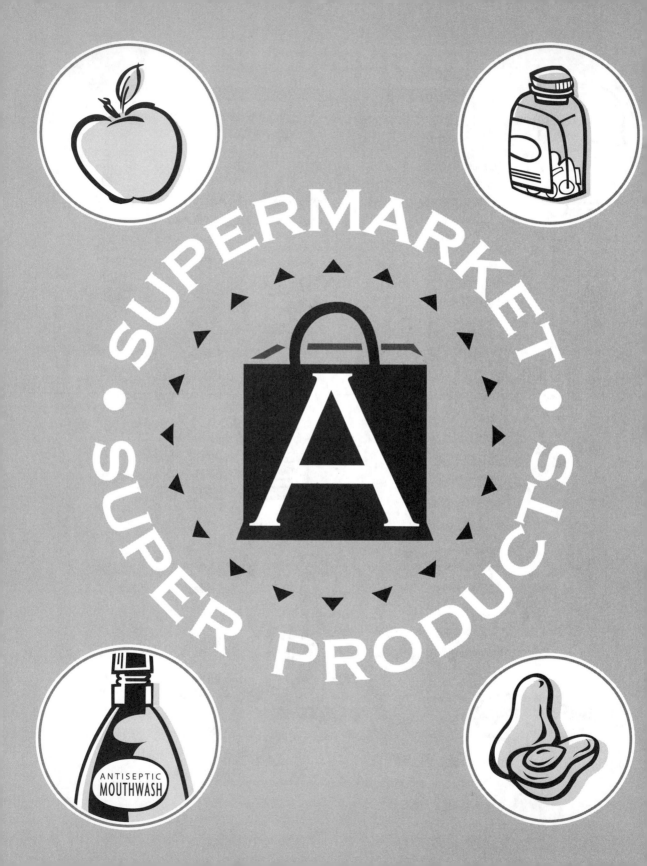

# ALCOHOL (RUBBING)

 ## Health & Beauty

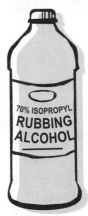

Here's a simple way to make a reusable ice pack: Mix 1 part rubbing alcohol with 2 parts water, and pour the solution into a heavy-duty plastic freezer bag (but don't fill it; leave room for expansion). Squeeze out all of the air, seal the bag, and put it in the freezer. Alcohol doesn't freeze, so the contents will be slushy rather than rock hard—and all the more comfortable on your achin' body.

Before using a needle to remove a splinter, wipe both your skin and the needle with rubbing alcohol to kill germs and prevent infection.

To cure swimmer's ear, mix equal parts of rubbing alcohol and vinegar, and pour the solution into the water-clogged ear. The alcohol will help dry up the trapped water, and the vinegar will kill any bacteria.

After you've pulled a tick out of your (or your pet's) skin, drop it into a jar of rubbing alcohol to kill it instantly. But don't dab the tick with alcohol—or anything else—before you pull it out. That can cause the varmint to regurgitate germs into the victim's skin.

**REMARKABLE RECIPES**

### AHHH AFTERSHAVE

Okay, guys—this one's for you. Here's an easy recipe that will make the women in your life go "Ahhh."

**2 cups of rubbing alcohol**
**1 tbsp. of glycerin**
**1 tbsp. of dried lavender**
**1 tsp. of dried rosemary**
**1 tsp. of ground cloves**

Mix all of the ingredients well, pour into a bottle with a tight-fitting cap, and refrigerate. Shake well before using, and strain as you use it. This aftershave will keep, refrigerated, for up to two months.

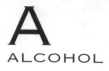

Had a run-in with poison ivy? If you act fast, you can lessen the effects of the rash, or even head it off. First, swab the affected skin with rubbing alcohol. It will cut through the plant's toxic oil and dilute it. Then wash the area with soap and water.

## Home Cleaning & Upkeep

Before you wash a grimy windowsill, wipe it with a soft cloth dipped in rubbing alcohol. It will dissolve the greasy dirt, so the detergent can really get in there and do its job.

After mopping your floor, disinfect the bucket by wiping it with rubbing alcohol on a rag.

To get wax buildup off of a floor, scrub it with a solution of 3 parts water to 1 part rubbing alcohol, and rinse thoroughly. (Make sure the room is well ventilated before you begin.)

Remove an ink spot from cloth by blotting the stain with rubbing alcohol, and laundering as usual.

When mustard oozes out of your hot dog bun and onto your shirt, reach for this mustard blaster: Scrub the spots with a solution of 2 parts water and 1 part rubbing alcohol, then toss the garment into the wash.

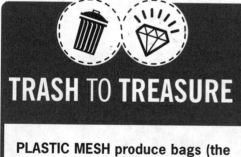

## TRASH TO TREASURE

PLASTIC MESH produce bags (the kind that onions and potatoes come in) make perfect bathroom scrubbers, whether you're using rubbing alcohol or any other cleanser. They won't scratch porcelain, tile, or marble surfaces, yet they're tough enough to clear off even the most stubborn grime like mildew and soap scum.

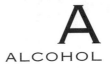

◆ Is your computer looking dingy? Grab some cotton balls, cotton swabs, and rubbing alcohol. It'll clean up the keyboard, mouse, and casing without leaving a soapy residue.

◆ Got nasty grass stains on your clothes? Before you wash the duds, scrub rubbing alcohol into the stains.

◆ Once a week, wipe your telephone receiver with a soft cloth dipped in rubbing alcohol. It will remove oils, grease, fingerprints, and ink stains—and kill cold-causing germs.

◆ Keep spiders outside where they belong by wiping windowsills with rubbing alcohol.

◆ When you clean your bathroom, give the fixtures a final rubdown with a little rubbing alcohol. It will kill germs, shine mirrors and chrome, and remove all traces of soap, deodorant, hair spray, and toothpaste.

◆ Get rid of mildew from caulking around tubs and showers by wiping the area with rubbing alcohol.

◆ Labels can leave sticky residue on glass. Wipe the area with rubbing alcohol to get rid of the goo.

## REMARKABLE RECIPES

## ONE-SHOT CLEANER

Here's a great recipe for a multipurpose cleaner.

**2 cups of rubbing alcohol**
**1 tbsp. of ammonia**
**1 tbsp. of dishwashing liquid**
**2 qt. of water**

Combine all of the ingredients, pour into a hand-held spray bottle, and go to town. (This super-duper concoction will beat commercial, streakless, glass-cleaning products hands down!)

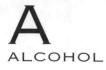

◆ Book covers mildewed? Sponge rubbing alcohol on the spots, and set the books in the sunlight until the splotches disappear.

◆ Here's an easy way to keep soap and mildew from building up on your tub, glass shower doors, or vinyl curtain liner. Just mix together 3 cups of water, ½ cup of rubbing alcohol, and 1 tablespoon of liquid laundry detergent that lists enzymes among its ingredients. Pour the solution into a hand-held spray bottle, and keep the bottle on the side of the tub. Then make a household rule that says, "The last person out of the shower or bath each day sprays the solution on all of the wet surfaces." Follow up once a month by wiping down the walls with the same solution, and you should never see mold or mildew again.

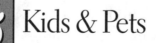

## Kids & Pets

■ Having trouble putting new rubber grips on a bike's handlebars? Rub some rubbing alcohol on the end of the handlebar, and the grip will slide right on.

■ If you find a great leather dog collar for peanuts at a tag sale, don't pass it up because it's a tad mildewed. You can get that leather looking as good as new by wiping the mildew away with a solution of equal parts rubbing alcohol and water. Follow up with a good leather conditioner.

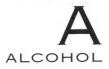

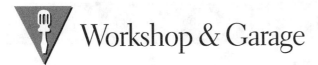

# Workshop & Garage

▼ You parked your car under a pine tree, and now it's covered with drops of sap. To get the sap off, dampen a soft cotton cloth with rubbing alcohol and buff the stuff away.

▼ Clean your car's chrome by rubbing it with a soft cloth dipped in rubbing alcohol.

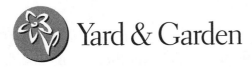

# Yard & Garden

● Want to get moss off of a brick or stone walkway? Spray the stuff with a solution of 2 tablespoons of rubbing alcohol per pint of water, then rinse it away with the garden hose.

● Rubbing alcohol is a potent weed killer. Just mix 2 tablespoons of alcohol with a pint of water, and pour the solution into a hand-held spray bottle. Drench each unwanted plant directly. Aim carefully, though, or you might kill off plants that you want to keep.

● Make a lethal insect spray by mixing 1 cup of rubbing alcohol and 1 teaspoon of vegetable oil in 1 quart of water in a hand-held spray bottle. Give each pest a direct hit.

● To kill mealybugs on your houseplants, dab each one with a cotton swab dipped in rubbing alcohol.

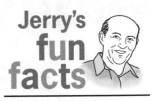

**Jerry's fun facts**

Do you know what the very first petrochemical was? It was good old rubbing (isopropyl) alcohol. Unlike many historic discoveries, though, this one did not happen by accident. In 1920, scientists at the Standard Oil Company in Linden, New Jersey, were trying hard to invent useful substances from by-products of gasoline manufacturing. They did a few clever procedures with propylene gas, and out came isopropyl alcohol.

# ALUMINUM FOIL

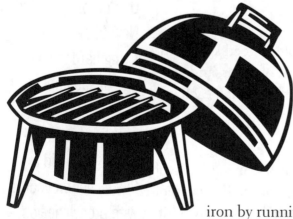

Aluminum Foil

## Home Cleaning & Upkeep

◆ To get cooked-on food off of cast-iron pots, ball up a piece of aluminum foil, and use it to rub the pan until the stains disappear. Wipe clean with a soft, dry cloth. (The same trick works with non-iron pans or casseroles—but in this case, boost the cleaning power with a little soap and water.)

◆ Want to speed up your ironing chores? Stretch a piece of aluminum foil over the ironing board, under the cover. It'll intensify the heat from the iron and make your job go faster.

◆ After your next barbecue, lay a sheet of aluminum foil on the hot grill. When it's cooled down, peel off the foil, crinkle it into a ball, and rub the grill clean. All those burned-on burgers will be gone faster than you can say, "Make mine medium rare."

◆ Clean starch off of an iron by running it over a piece of aluminum foil.

◆ When you've used a steel-wool soap pad for light duty, don't throw it away—wrap it in aluminum foil, and tuck it in the freezer. It'll live to clean another day!

◆ Got a vinyl floor tile that won't stay put? Place a piece of aluminum foil on top of the tile, and run a hot iron over it several times to melt the glue underneath. Then set a pile of books or magazines on top of the tile until the glue dries completely.

◆ Clean up oxidation pits on unpainted aluminum doors and windows by wadding up a ball of aluminum foil and rubbing it back and forth across the pitted areas. This won't make the oxidation disappear, but little bits of the foil will catch in the pits and make your door or window look better, at least for the short haul.

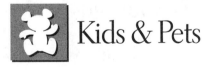

## Kids & Pets

■ To keep Fido and Fluffy off of the furniture, lay sheets of aluminum foil on the seat cushions. The rustling sound and the strange feel will send them seeking comfort elsewhere.

■ Try this cat-pleaser: Wad up some aluminum foil into a 1½-inch ball. Presto!—instant feline fun!

**REMARKABLE RECIPES**

## SUPER SILVER CLEANING FORMULA

Here's the easiest recipe I know of for getting tarnished silver bright and shiny again.

**Aluminum foil**

**2 pans that can hold enough water to cover your silver pieces**

**1 cup of baking soda per gal. of water**

**Water**

Line the bottom of one pan with foil, and set in your tarnished treasure. Make sure the silver touches the aluminum (I say this in case there's a non-silver part to the object). Then fill the second pan with water and heat it to boiling. Remove the pan from the heat, set it in the sink, and add the baking soda. Be careful—the solution will foam up and may spill over. Pour the soda solution into the first pan, completely covering the silver. Within seconds, you'll see the tarnish start to disappear. A lightly tarnished piece should be clean as a whistle in 4 or 5 minutes; one with a heavy coat of tarnish may need a few more treatments.

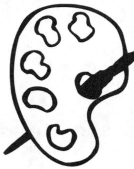

■ In a battery-powered toy, a broken spring can spell disaster. But aluminum foil can spell relief. Just wedge a small piece of foil between the battery and the spring. The result: a real power play! (This same trick works with portable radios and other small appliances.)

■ Your youngster has suddenly turned into a junior Georgia O'Keefe, and she needs a paint palette, *pronto!* No problem—just wrap aluminum foil around a sheet of heavy cardboard.

■ Want to keep the kids busy indoors on a cold winter day? Have them make Christmas tree ornaments by tracing cookie-cutter shapes onto cardboard, cutting them out, and covering them with foil, shiny side out. (These bright bangles are also great for scaring birds away from your fruit trees and berry bushes.)

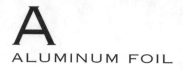

## Jerry's fun facts

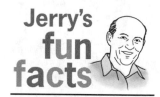

Every year, folks in the United States use 500 million pounds of aluminum foil and foil containers. That adds up to 8 million miles of foil – enough to stretch from earth to the moon and back about 18 times!

## Workshop & Garage

▼ No time to clean your paintbrushes? Wrap them (still wet) in aluminum foil and stash them in the freezer. When you're ready to paint again, defrost the brushes for an hour or so, and they'll be good to go.

▼ To keep a crust from forming on leftover paint, try this simple trick: Set the paint can on a sheet of aluminum foil, and trace around the bottom of the can. Then cut out the foil disk, lay it on the paint surface, and close up the can.

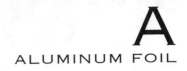

▼ Before you start to paint, mold foil around any hardware that you don't want to get paint on, such as doorknobs, drawer pulls, and coat hooks.

▼ Here's an old-time solution for removing rust from your car's chrome. Crumple up a piece of aluminum foil so that the shiny side is facing out, and scrub the rusty spots. For really stubborn stains, pour a little cola onto the foil. Those spots will disappear like a quarter in a magician's hand.

▼ Need a one-time funnel for a really grimy job? Lay a sheet of aluminum foil over a sheet of newspaper, fold in half, and roll it all into the shape of a cone.

 ## Yard & Garden

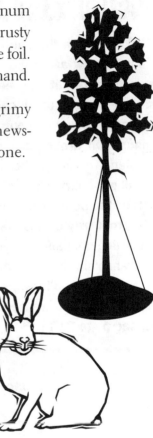

● To guard young trees from mice and rabbits, wrap the trunks loosely in aluminum foil to a height of 18 inches to 2 feet. The glittering, rattling surface will send the gnawers looking elsewhere for food.

● Got herbs or geraniums spending the cold months on indoor windowsills? Line the sills with aluminum foil, shiny side up. It'll reflect light onto the plants and keep them going strong all winter long. To increase the light level even more, cover a panel of cardboard with foil, and hang it on a wall so that it reflects the light from a window onto your potted plants. Besides boosting their growth, it'll keep them evenly shaped.

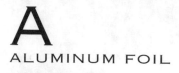

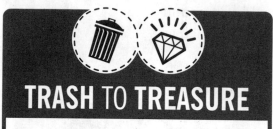

## TRASH TO TREASURE

**WHEN YOU reach the end of a roll of foil, don't throw away the cardboard tube. Instead, turn it into seed-starting pots. Just cut it into pieces about 3 inches long, and wrap (you guessed it) aluminum foil around the outside of each piece to keep the cardboard from falling apart when it gets wet. Pack the little pots closely together on a waterproof tray or shallow pan, add seed-starting mix, and sow your seeds. Come transplant time, remove the foil, and plant your seedlings, pots and all. (For another way to reuse cardboard tubes, see page 213.)**

● Want to force bulbs, but lack the refrigerator space to give them the chilly darkness they need? Here's your answer: Put the bulbs on a cold windowsill, and cover them with a cone of aluminum foil. Remove the foil when crocus shoots reach 2 inches or when hyacinth shoots reach 4 inches tall.

● Protect tender transplants from cutworms by wrapping aluminum foil loosely around each stem. The foil should extend about 2 inches below the ground and 3 inches above.

● Use aluminum foil mulch to speed plants' growth and increase production. Just stretch the foil on the ground between plants, and anchor it along the edges with stones or bricks. Light reflecting off the foil can increase yields, especially in cloudy weather, and speed the ripening of tomatoes or the blooming of a rosebush by a full two weeks!

● Aluminum foil placed on the soil around plants will also deter aphids, thrips, moths, and other flying insects. How? The light bouncing off the foil confuses the bugs so much that they can't land.

● Brighten the lights in your yard or campsite by giving each lamp a reflective backdrop. Just wrap pieces of wood or cardboard in foil, shiny side up, and set one behind each light.

# AMMONIA

 ## Health & Beauty

Take the itch and swelling out of a mosquito bite by dabbing the spot with a few drops of ammonia. Make sure that you use this treatment *before* you start scratching. If the skin is already broken, the ammonia will deliver a sting you won't soon forget!

To bleach the hair on your upper lip, mix ¼ cup of hydrogen peroxide (6 percent) with 1 teaspoon of ammonia. Dip a cotton ball into the solution, and dab it onto the hair. Let it sit for 30 minutes, then rinse it off with cool water.

## Home Cleaning & Upkeep

Do you have an oven that's not self-cleaning? To do the job yourself the easy way, combine ¼ cup of ammonia and 2 cups of water in a glass baking dish. Put the dish in the oven, shut the door, and leave it overnight. In the morning, the grime will wipe away easily with a sponge.

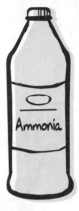

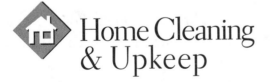

### NO-RINSE, ALL-PURPOSE CLEANER

Who needs expensive, "miracle" spray cleaners? This natural recipe cleans floors, woodwork, greasy countertops, and appliances, and even kills mildew. What's more, you don't even need to rinse!

**1 cup of clear ammonia**
**½ cup of white vinegar**
**¼ cup of baking soda**
**1 gal. of hot water**

Mix all of the ingredients in a bucket. Then pour the solution into a hand-held spray bottle, or sponge it on straight from the pail.

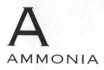

◆ Don't cry over spilled milk! Instead, clean it (or ice cream) off of your upholstery this way: First, scrub the area gently with a mixture of dishwashing liquid and warm water. Follow up with a solution of 2 tablespoons of ammonia to 4 cups of water. Wash the spot again with dishwashing liquid and water. Finally, saturate a clean cotton cloth with warm water, wring it out, and scrub gently. Then let the spot dry naturally.

◆ If your moo-juice stains are on a wooden surface, don't have a cow! Put a few drops of ammonia on a dampened cloth, and rub gently. The milk should come right out.

◆ You forgot you had clothes in the washer and they turned "sour" before you could dry them? Put them through the wash cycle again, but this time with a tablespoon or so of ammonia—no detergent—to freshen them up.

◆ Has a plastic bread bag melted on the outside of your toaster oven? First, unplug the oven and let it cool down. Then cover the plastic with a cloth soaked in ammonia. Wait 3 or 4 minutes, and scrape the stuff off with a plastic scraper or plastic scouring pad.

◆ To clean glass tabletops, spray them with a solution of 2 tablespoons of ammonia to 1 quart of water. Dry with a soft cotton cloth. If the glass is surrounded by wood, spray the solution in the center of the glass and work slowly toward the edges—and be careful not to get any of the cleaner on the wood.

◆ We all know that TV and computer screens are real dust and dirt magnets. To keep them squeaky-clean, mix ¼ cup of ammonia in 2 quarts of warm water. Dip a soft cotton cloth or sponge in the solution, and apply it sparingly to the screen.

◆ To polish pewter, wipe it with a soft cotton cloth dipped in a solution of 2 tablespoons of ammonia to 1 quart of hot soapy water.

◆ If squirrels have set up housekeeping in your chimney, pour a little ammonia in a pan, and set it on the hearth. Just make sure that the flue is open and the fumes can travel up the chimney. I guarantee that the critters will scurry in a hurry!

# Workshop & Garage

▼ To clean your windshield-wiper blades, pull each wiper away from the windshield and rub down both sides with a rag soaked in ammonia.

▼ Car headlights can get *really* grimy, especially in the winter. To get them sparkling clean, use a solution of 2 tablespoons of ammonia to 1 quart of water, and mix in a tablespoon of cornstarch, which will act as a mild abrasive. Then rinse the headlights with clear water.

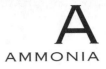

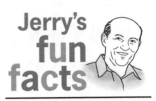

**Jerry's fun facts**

Have you ever wondered exactly what ammonia is? I'll tell you: It's a compound of 1 part nitrogen to 3 parts hydrogen, and the fellow who discovered how to make it — a German chemist named Fritz Haber — won a Nobel prize for his efforts in 1918. But that's not the end of the glory story. Another German chemist, Carl Bosch, refined the process so that ammonia could be made commercially. That bit of brainwork earned him a Nobel prize, too, in 1931.

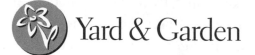 Yard & Garden

● To force cut branches of flowering shrubs, such as lilac or forsythia, into bloom, set the stems in a bucket of warm water. Drop in a cotton ball soaked with ammonia, and cover both the branches and the bucket with a plastic bag.

● If you're starting seeds indoors, and the containers have been used before, wash each one in a mild solution of 8 parts soapy water to 1 part ammonia before you fill the pot with sterilized potting mix.

● Ants will vamoose if you pour ammonia down their hill, and follow up with boiling water.

● Practically all four-legged garden pests—including gophers, groundhogs, skunks, squirrels, and roaming pets—will flee from the scent of ammonia. Just soak rags in the stuff, put them in old pantyhose toes, and hang them in the areas you want to protect. If there's no hanging space, pour the ammonia into wide-necked bottles, like the kind juice comes in, and bury them up to the rims.

● Ammonia is a super slug killer. Pour ½ cup into a spray bottle, add 1 tablespoon of Murphy's Oil Soap® and 1½ cups of water, and shake well.

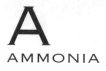

### LAWN FRESH-UP TONIC

How do you know when to water your grass? Simple: Walk on it. If it doesn't spring right back up, it's thirsty. To help the water go straight to the roots, put on your golf shoes or a pair of aerating lawn sandals, and take a stroll around your yard. Then follow up with this tonic.

**1 can of beer**
**1 cup of baby shampoo**
**½ cup of ammonia**
**½ cup of weak tea**

Mix all of these ingredients in your 20 gallon hose-end sprayer, and apply to the point of run-off.

# ANTACID TABLETS

 ## Health & Beauty

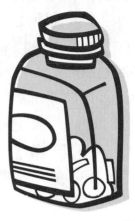

● Quitting smoking? Great! As long as you're not on a low-sodium diet and don't have ulcers, drink two antacid tablets (like Alka-Seltzer®) dissolved in a glass of water at each meal to help curb your nicotine cravings.

● Soothe bug bites by dissolving two antacid tablets in a glass of water. Then moisten a soft cloth with the solution, and hold it on the bite for 20 minutes.

 ## Home Cleaning & Upkeep

◆ Drop a couple of antacid tablets (like Alka-Seltzer®) into your toilet. Wait 20 minutes, then brush and flush. That bowl will come out sparkling clean!

◆ Unclog a drain by dropping in three antacid tablets followed by a cup of white vinegar. Give them a few minutes to work before running the hot water for 3 to 4 minutes.

◆ Remove stains from the bottom of vases and cruets by filling them with water and dropping in a couple of antacid tablets.

# A

ANTACID TABLETS

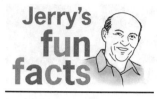
In 1928, Hub Beardsley, the president of Miles Laboratories, visited an Indiana newspaper at the height of a flu epidemic. Many of Mr. Beardsley's employees were out sick, yet not one person on the paper's staff had missed a single day of work. How come? Because, at the first sign of flu symptoms, the paper's editor dosed his troops with aspirin and baking soda. Mr. Beardsley took the idea back to his laboratory, had his head chemist whip it up in tablet form, and — plop, plop, fizz, fizz — Alka-Seltzer® was born!

◆ To polish your jewelry, use two antacid tablets in a glass of water. Let the pieces soak for 2 minutes, then rinse them in cool water. (But don't use this treatment on pearls or opals.)

◆ Thermos® bottle smelling stale? Fill it with water and drop in four antacid tablets. Let it sit for an hour, and rinse thoroughly. It'll come out clean and fresh as new.

◆ Get a ceramic sink sparkling clean by filling with 2 to 3 inches of water, then dropping in two antacid tablets. Wait 20 minutes or so, then drain the sink and give it a wipedown with a damp sponge.

◆ Burned grease inside your pots and pans? Fill 'em with water, and drop in six antacid tablets. Let them soak for an hour, and wash as usual.

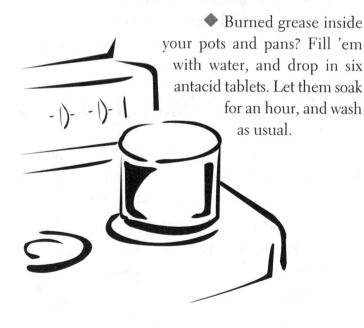

# ANTISEPTIC MOUTHWASH

## Health & Beauty

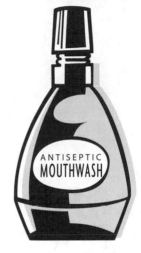

Fresh out of deodorant? Dab a little antiseptic mouthwash under your arms. It'll kill the bacteria that cause odor.

Pour antiseptic mouthwash over cuts and scrapes. It kills germs on your skin as well as in your mouth.

When mosquito bites have you itching like crazy, reach for a bottle of antiseptic mouthwash. Moisten a tissue with it, hold it on the bite for about 15 seconds, and kiss that itch goodbye!

Prevent dandruff by washing your hair with antiseptic mouthwash every two weeks or so.

## Home Cleaning & Upkeep

You never know who's been washing what at a laundromat. Set your mind at ease by wiping the washer's surface with antiseptic mouthwash. Then, to disinfect the innards, add ½ cup of mouthwash to the wash cycle.

Keep high-chair trays, table tops, and baby teething toys germ-free by wiping them down with antiseptic mouthwash.

# A

◆ Antiseptic mouthwash kills germs anywhere. If something's smelling up the fridge, or you need to clean the toilet bowl and you're fresh out of other cleansers, just reach for the mouthwash, pour some onto a sponge, and have at it!

◆ Before you hang wallpaper, spray the damp, pasted side with antiseptic mouthwash. It'll keep mildew from growing in the paste and discoloring the paper.

 Yard & Garden

● To fend off root rot all through your garden, add plenty of organic matter to the soil to ensure good drainage, and douse your plants' roots in early spring with a solution of ½ cup of antiseptic mouthwash and ½ cup of baby shampoo per 2 gallons of warm water.

● Feed your lawn with this mixture: 1 cup of antiseptic mouthwash, 1 cup of Epsom salts, 1 cup of dishwashing liquid, and 1 cup of ammonia in your 20 gallon hose-end sprayer. Fill the balance of the sprayer jar with warm water, and let 'er rip.

● After you prune trees, seal the wounds with a mixture of antiseptic mouthwash and latex paint.

## REMARKABLE RECIPES

## TREE WOUND STERILIZER TONIC

Anytime you cut diseased tissue from a tree or shrub, kill lingering germs with this powerful potion.

**¼ cup of antiseptic mouthwash**
**¼ cup of ammonia**
**¼ cup of dishwashing liquid**
**1 gal. of warm water**

Mix all of the ingredients, pour the solution into a hand-held spray bottle, and drench the places where you've pruned off limbs or branches.

# APPLES & APPLE JUICE

 Health & Beauty

🍎 Here's a simple facial formula that will slough off dead skin cells, refine pores, and even out your skin tone. In a small bowl, mix 2 teaspoons of apple juice, 2 teaspoons of red wine, and 1 tablespoon of ground oatmeal to make a paste. (Add more liquid if you need to.) Spread the mixture onto your face and throat, let it dry for 20 to 30 minutes, and rinse with warm water.

🍎 Got garlicky breath? Chase it away by biting into an apple, then brushing your teeth.

🍎 To ease the discomfort of constipation, mix ½ cup of applesauce with four to six chopped prunes and 1 tablespoon of bran. Eat this concoction just before bed, and by morning, things should be on the move again!

🍎 Although it may seem odd, applesauce can solve the opposite problem, too. The anti-diarrhea formula is 1 teaspoon of carob powder in ¼ cup of applesauce. Eat it slowly, and take up to two or three doses throughout the day.

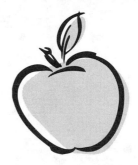

**REMARKABLE RECIPES**

## APPLE ASTRINGENT

The acids in apple juice tone your skin and help keep it clear—and they're mild enough to use on even sensitive skin.

**½ cup of apple juice**
**4 tbsp. of vodka (100 proof)**
**1 tbsp. of honey**
**1 tsp. of sea salt**

Pour all of the ingredients into a bottle with a tight cap, and shake well. Apply the solution to your face and neck twice a day with a cotton pad.

## Home Cleaning & Upkeep

◆ A slice of apple will soften hard brown sugar. Just tuck the chunk into the bag, and in a day or so, the sugar will be as good as new.

◆ Here's an old-time way to remove a broken light bulb that's still in the socket. *First, make sure the power to the fixture is turned off.* Next, push half of an apple onto the glass, with the cut side up against the broken bulb. Turn the apple just as you would to unscrew a whole light bulb. Once it's out of the socket, don't try to remove the bulb from the apple—just toss it all in the trash. (You can also use half a potato for this trick.)

◆ Got an aluminum pan that's discolored? Fill it with enough water to cover the stains, toss in some apple peels, and boil it for a few minutes. Rinse and dry, and it'll be as good as new!

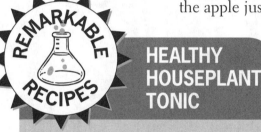

### HEALTHY HOUSEPLANT TONIC

To keep your houseplants in the pink of health, feed them with this elixir.

**1 can of apple juice**
**1 can of beer**
**1 can of regular cola (not diet)**
**1 cup of lemon-scented dishwashing liquid**
**1 cup of lemon-scented ammonia**
**½ cup of Fish Emulsion**

Mix all of these ingredients in a big old pot. Store the solution in a covered container, and use 3 ounces per gallon of water every other time you water your houseplants.

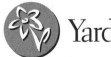 ## Yard & Garden

● Flowering shrubs love apples. To keep those bloomers purring right along, bury all your apple peels and over-the-hill fruit in the soil around your shrubs.

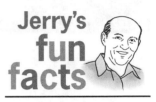

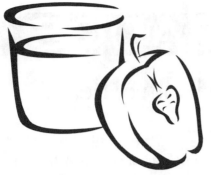

● Apple juice is a great tonic for all kinds of plants. Mix 1 cup of juice with 10 gallons of water, and spray the solution on lawns, flowers, shrubs, and trees.

● To make your groundcover thick enough to stop a jackrabbit, apply this top-dressing recipe: Mix 10 parts worm castings with 5 parts ground apple, and add to ½ bushel of compost. Then overspray everything with my Flower Feeder Tonic (see page 43).

● When Old Man Winter is coming in fast and your garden is still full of unripe veggies, pour 1 cup of apple juice, ½ cup of ammonia, and ½ cup of baby shampoo into your 20 gallon hose-end sprayer. Fill the balance of the jar with warm water, and spray your plants to the point of run-off.

● Are maggots spoiling your apple crop? Foil 'em with apples. Here's how: Before the blossoms on your trees turn to fruit, buy some red apples with the stems still attached. (You'll need two for a dwarf tree; six to eight for a full-sized one.) Coat the apples with corn syrup or spray them with a commercial adhesive, and hang them in your trees. The adult flies will zero in on the apples to lay their eggs, and get stuck in the stick-um.

**Jerry's fun facts**

We all learned about Johnny Appleseed in our gradeschool days. You probably will remember that his real name was Jonathan Chapman, and you may recall that he grew up in what is now Arlington, Massachusetts. But here's something I'll bet you don't know: One of Johnny's boyhood pals was another budding folk hero, Samuel Wilson, better known in his later years as Uncle Sam—the real-life inspiration for one of our country's most beloved symbols.

# A

# AVOCADOS

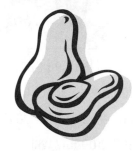

## ✚ Health & Beauty

❦ Does your hair have a case of the dry frizzies? Get things under control with an avocado. Simply skin and mash a ripe avocado, work it into your hair, and leave it on for 15 minutes. Rinse it out with cool water and—holy guacamole—your hair will be moist, shiny, and frizz-free!

❦ If you live in a place where your hair has to face heat, smog, and fog, this deep conditioner is just for you. First, mash ½ of an avocado with ¼ cup of mayonnaise (the real stuff, with eggs and oil in it). Massage the mixture into your scalp, and comb it out to the ends of your hair. Cover your hair with a shower cap, and wrap a hot, wet towel around your head. Leave it on for at least 30 minutes, and then rinse.

❦ For a softening and invigorating facial, try this: Combine 2 tablespoons of mashed avocado, 1 tablespoon of crushed almonds, and ½ teaspoon of honey, and stir until creamy. Apply the mixture to your skin, and leave it on for 30 minutes or so. Rinse with warm water, and pat dry.

## REMARKABLE RECIPES

### FACE FOOD

You would be hard-pressed to find a more skin-pleasing fruit than an avocado. Its high fat content makes it the perfect base for a nourishing facial masque.

**½ of an avocado**
**1 tbsp. of plain yogurt**
**½ tsp. of vitamin E oil**

Mash the avocado, then blend in the yogurt and vitamin E. Smooth the mixture onto your face, paying close attention to the fine lines around your eyes and mouth. Leave the masque on for 20 minutes, and rinse it off with warm water.

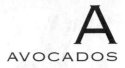

Here's an even easier facial masque. The next time you eat an avocado, save the peel, and leave some of the fruit on it. Then rub the peel over your face. The gritty texture of the rind sloughs off dead skin, while the fruit that stays on your face moisturizes it. Leave the green stuff in place for 10 minutes, and rinse with cool water. (This is also the perfect recipe for using up those too-ripe avocados you found in the bottom of the crisper drawer in your fridge!)

 Yard & Garden

Avocados are a potent source of potassium and magnesium. Just bury the peels near your flowering plants (especially roses), then stand back, and watch the show. If you have leftover avocado chunks that haven't been doused with dressing, use them, too!

Use avocado skins as slug traps. Set them out before dark, and slugs will slither in overnight. Come morning, scoop up your traps, and drop them into a bucket of soapy water. Then toss it all on the compost pile.

## TRASH TO TREASURE

**DON'T THROW** away your avocado pits (at least not all of them): You can turn them into lush, green houseplants. Just peel off the brown covering, and stick three toothpicks into the middle of the seed so that you can suspend it, flat end down, over a jar of water. The bottom of the pit should just touch the water. Place the glass in a dark, warm spot. As the water evaporates, add more to keep the bottom of the pit wet. In four to eight weeks, you'll see roots. Soon after that, a green stem and leaves will appear. When that happens, plant the seed in a container filled with commercial potting soil, and move it to a sunny location. As your seedling grows, keep pinching back the growing tip, and turn the pot around now and then, so your plant will grow bushy and even. When warm weather comes, be sure to move your plant outdoors. It will thrive in the heat, and summers in the sun will make it grow by leaps and bounds!

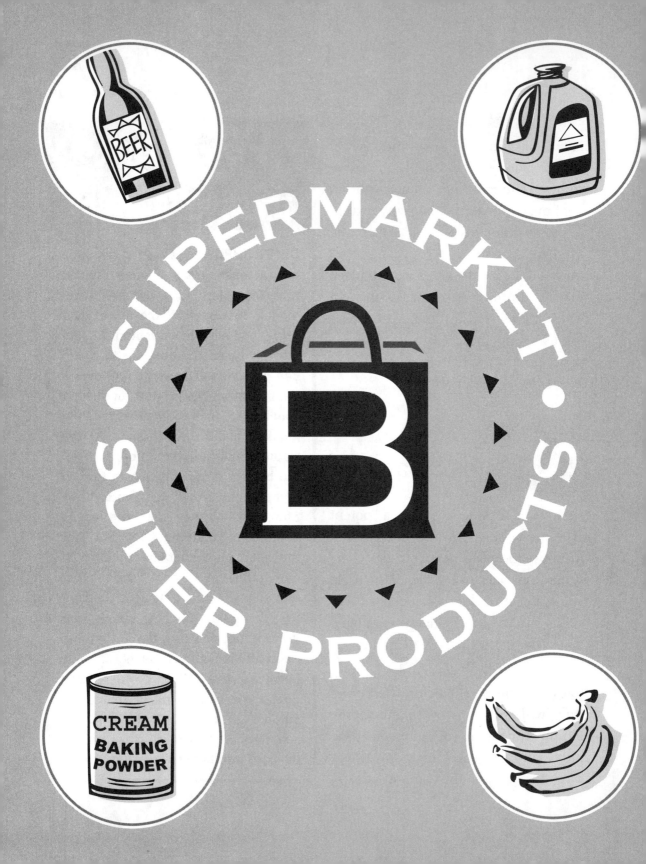

# BABY OIL

 ## Health & Beauty

 Mascara dry and clumpy? Drip a drop of baby oil into the tube, insert the brush, and twirl it around. *Voilà*—no more clumps!

 A drop or two of baby oil in your bath water will leave your skin feeling soft and fresh. But, be careful getting out of the tub—the oil may make it slippery.

 Out of makeup remover or cold cream? Put a little baby oil on a cotton ball and use that instead—but be careful around your eyes.

 When your lips are cracked and dry—or you just want a little gloss—rub on a small amount of baby oil.

 Got an adhesive bandage stuck to your skin? Don't tug and pull at it. Instead, soak a cotton ball in baby oil and apply to the bandage. It'll come right off.

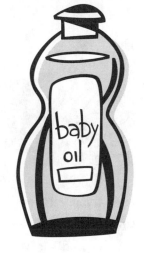

 ## Home Cleaning & Upkeep

◆ Keep soap scum from forming on your shower doors by giving them a good rubdown with a few drops of baby oil on a soft, clean cloth or sponge. Don't use too much, though, or you'll end up with a greasy mess!

◆ Can't get that knot out of your jewelry chain? Put a drop of baby oil on the knot to loosen it, and then patiently work it out with a couple of safety pins or sewing needles. (Magnifying eyeglasses sure come in handy for this job!)

◆ Baby oil is a great chrome polish. Wipe it on with a soft, clean cloth to make all of the chrome around your home or on your car bright and shiny.

## REMARKABLE RECIPES

### HOMEMADE BABY WIPES

Why buy expensive baby wipes, when you've probably got everything you need to make your own? Here's how it's done.

**1 roll of soft, absorbent paper towels (premium brands work best)**

**1 plastic container with a tight-fitting lid to hold the paper towels**

**2 tbsp. of baby oil**

**2 tbsp. of liquid baby bath soap**

**2 cups of water**

Cut the roll of paper towels in half with a serrated knife, and remove the cardboard tube. Place half the roll, on end, in the plastic container. Mix the liquid ingredients, pour the solution into the container, and close the lid. The towels will absorb the liquid. As you need them, pull the wipes up from the center of the roll.

## Kids & Pets

◆ Before you take Fido for a stroll on messy wintertime sidewalks, wipe baby oil into the hair between his toes. It will make dirt, salt, and snow-melting chemicals easier to wash off.

◆ Planning on showing off your pet chickens at the county fair? Then soften the dry or rough skin on their feet with a little baby oil.

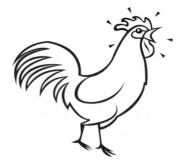

# BABY POWDER

 Health & Beauty

 For a dry shampoo that will leave your hair clean and fresh-smelling, rub baby powder through the strands, then brush it out.

 When it comes to softening hands, baby powder works wonders. Just smooth it on as you would lotion.

 If you want your favorite grownup bath powder to last longer, mix some baby powder in with it.

 When a day at the beach leaves you with damp, sandy skin from head to toe, sprinkle yourself with baby powder. It'll absorb the moisture, and the sand will all but fall off.

 Do you shave your legs with an electric razor? Dust them with baby powder first to prevent friction burns.

 Home Cleaning & Upkeep

 To keep your shoes (especially hard-working sneakers) dry, comfortable, and fresh-smelling, dust the insides with baby powder.

**REMARKABLE RECIPES**

## CREAM DEODORANT

This simple concoction will keep you as fresh and dry as any store-bought brand.

**2 tbsp. of baby powder**
**2 tbsp. of baking soda**
**2 tbsp. of petroleum jelly**

Combine all of these ingredients in a pan, and heat over low heat until the mixture is smooth and creamy. Store it in an airtight container until you're ready to use it.

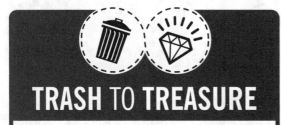

◆ When the weather turns hot and steamy, sprinkle baby powder on your sheets to absorb perspiration and prevent stuck-in-bed syndrome.

◆ When a chain necklace seems hopelessly tangled, loosen it up with a sprinkling of baby powder.

◆ A white shirt won't absorb oily grime (particularly around the neck) if you sprinkle it with baby powder before you iron it.

◆ Hide a stain on a white suit or coat by rubbing baby powder into the spot.

◆ Got grease splattered on the wall? Pour baby powder onto a soft cotton cloth, and rub the spots until they disappear.

## TRASH TO TREASURE

AFTER YOU'VE emptied a baby powder container, wash it out, and turn it into a mini sprinkling can. It's perfect for giving houseplants a gentle shower, and it's just the ticket for tiny tots who want to help water the garden.

## Yard & Garden

● To keep squirrels and other rodents away from your bulbs, dust the bulbs with medicated baby powder before planting them.

● When you dig up tender bulbs for winter storage, give them a dose of medicated baby powder. It'll fend off rot and other fungal woes.

● Discourage deer from feasting on your young trees and shrubs by sprinkling baby powder on rags and hanging them among the branches.

# BABY WIPES

 ## Health & Beauty

🍎 Because baby wipes are gentle enough for babies, they're perfect to use on grownup skin after an operation—even on the most sensitive areas of your body. (If you have stitches or any broken skin, check with your doctor first.)

🍎 Baby those painful hemorrhoids by using baby wipes instead of toilet tissue. Be sure to toss them in the trash—baby wipes aren't flushable!

🍎 Clean scrapes and minor abrasions with baby wipes.

🍎 Use baby wipes to remove makeup. (Keep them away from your eyes, though!)

## Home Cleaning & Upkeep

◆ Blot up spilled coffee or other liquids from a carpet with baby wipes. They'll absorb the mess without leaving a stain.

◆ Tired of folks tracking into the house with dirty shoes? Keep a box of baby wipes by the door and ask everybody to clean up before they come inside.

◆ Remove crayon marks from walls by scrubbing them with a baby wipe.

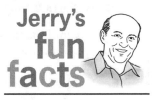

## Jerry's fun facts

Do you buy baby wipes even though you don't have a baby? You're not alone. Marketing studies show that 36% of the baby wipes sold in supermarkets are bought by folks whose children are more than 4 years old, or who don't even have any children!

# B

BABY WIPES

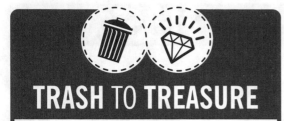
## Workshop & Garage

▼ Got something greasy on your car? Reach for a baby wipe: It'll clean up the mess without harming your car's paint job.

▼ Now and then, rub a baby wipe over your hammers, screwdrivers, and other tools. It'll keep them clean and free of rust.

▼ Clean your car's vinyl or cloth upholstery (but not leather!) by rubbing it with baby wipes. Use the unscented kind if you don't want your car's interior to smell like a nursery.

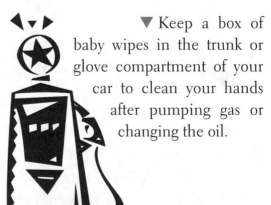

▼ Keep a box of baby wipes in the trunk or glove compartment of your car to clean your hands after pumping gas or changing the oil.

# BAKING POWDER

 ## Health & Beauty

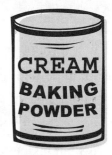

Do your feet tend to sweat? If so, then rub them with a little baking powder before you put your socks on. They'll stay dry and fresh as a daisy!

When the temperature climbs and you're fresh out of deodorant, brush on some baking powder.

Baking powder makes a fine substitute for face powder. (Just don't overdo it, or you'll look like Clarabel the Clown.)

## Home Cleaning & Upkeep

If your wallpaper is too delicate for commercial cleansers, make a paste of baking powder and water. Apply it with a sponge to remove any smudges and stains.

Before you pull on rubber gloves, pour a little baking powder into them. They'll be easier to remove when your chores are through.

When oil spills onto a rug, you need to clean it up *pronto*, before it has a chance to sink in and become a permanent fixture. Sprinkle baking powder on the spot to absorb the greasy mess. Let it dry, then vacuum the residue away.

# B
## BAKING POWDER

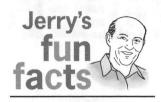
◆ Got a musty old trunk? First, take it outside into the fresh air and sunlight. Then pour a thin layer of baking powder in the bottom, and close it up. Sweep out the old powder and add a fresh supply every few days until the musty odor disappears.

◆ To de-mustify books or other small objects, put them in a bag with baking powder. Change it every few days until the aroma is gone.

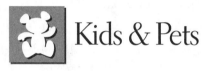 ## Kids & Pets

■ Fresh out of baby powder? Reach for the baking powder—it makes a perfect stand-in.

■ Baking powder sprinkled on bed linens will prevent heat rash in youngsters (or anyone else, for that matter).

■ Fluffy needs a bath, but she has a fit at the sight of water. What to do? Give her a dry bath: Just rub baking powder into her fur, then brush it out. Presto—a clean *and* happy (or, at least, content) kitty!

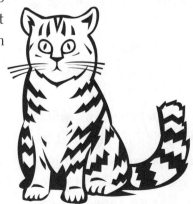

# BAKING SODA

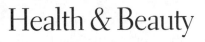 Health & Beauty

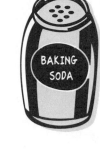

One of the easiest ways to soothe a bite or sting is to mix up a thick paste made from lukewarm water and baking soda, and apply it to the area (*after* you get the stinger out).

Cure indigestion fast by drinking a solution of a teaspoon of baking soda in a glass of water. The alkaline properties of the soda (a.k.a. sodium bicarbonate) will neutralize the overactive acids in your stomach.

Get your hairbrushes and combs nice and clean in a solution of baking soda and hot water.

For the power of a deep-cleaning beauty salon shampoo, add a little baking soda to your regular shampoo every week or so. Your hair will be cleaner and more manageable (without the beauty salon price tag).

Get rid of odors on your hands by adding a little baking soda to the soapy water when you scrub them.

Add 2 teaspoons of baking soda to a bowl of water to clean dentures or retainers.

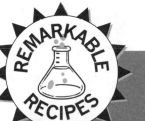

## PERFECT PEPPERMINT TOOTHPASTE

This mouth pleaser will leave your teeth sparklin' clean and your breath kissin' sweet.

**1 tbsp. of baking soda**
**¼ tsp. of peppermint extract (available in the supermarket spice section)**
**Dash of salt**

Combine the ingredients until you've got a toothpaste-like consistency. Then brush, and enjoy!

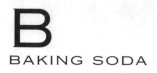

Soak in a warm bath with ½ cup of baking soda to ease the itch and pain of sunburn, chicken pox, or bug bites.

Got tired, achy feet? Soak those tootsies in a basin of hot water with ¼ cup of baking soda mixed in.

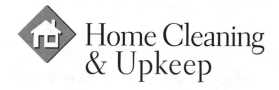

## Home Cleaning & Upkeep

Here's a natural way to sweeten and freshen any load of laundry. Add ½ cup of baking soda to the wash cycle and the same amount of white vinegar to the rinse cycle. Use more if you have hard water.

Mix a pinch or two of baking soda with water to wash pesticide residue from fresh-picked (or store-bought) fruits and vegetables.

Baking soda will remove tough grease and grime from appliances like your refrigerator or stovetop. Just dampen a sponge with hot water, and sprinkle some baking soda on the sponge. Scrub lightly, then rinse.

For really stubborn stains on porcelain sinks and tubs, make a paste of baking soda and water, let it sit for an hour or two, and then rinse.

Keep your dishwasher clean and odor-free: Once a month, fill the soap dispenser with baking soda (no soap) and run the empty machine through a full cycle.

◆ Contrary to its name, stainless steel *can* be stained by tea and any number of foods. Banish the marks using a paste made of 3 parts baking soda to 1 part water.

◆ Vomit, whether from pets or humans, is highly acidic. To clean it off of carpets or upholstery, sprinkle baking soda on the spots to neutralize the acid and deodorize the area. Use a plastic scraper to pick up the clumps that form, then vacuum the rest away.

◆ To clean and deodorize a wooden cutting board, mix equal parts of baking soda and salt with enough water to make a paste. Scrub this concoction into the board, leave it on for a few hours, and then rinse thoroughly.

◆ Everybody knows that an open box of baking soda keeps a refrigerator smelling fresh. Well, it can do the same for kitchen, bathroom, and basement cupboards, clothes closets, babies' rooms, and anyplace else where unpleasant odors tend to gather. Just remember to replace the box every two months or so.

◆ To freshen places where a box of baking soda won't fit, just sprinkle a little soda on the surface. It'll keep odor-catchers like mattresses, clothes hampers, and garbage cans less aromatic. (Sprinkle some inside shoes and sneakers to deodorize them, too.)

## REMARKABLE RECIPES

## SAFE & SOUND DRAIN CLEANER

Use this unclogger once a month to keep your drains open and clean-smelling—without corroding your plumbing or burning your skin.

**⅓ cup of baking soda**
**⅓ cup of table salt**
**1 tbsp. of cream of tartar**
**1 cup of boiling water**

Combine the soda, salt, and cream of tartar, and pour the mixture into the drain. Immediately add 1 cup of boiling water. Wait 10 seconds, then flush with cold water for at least 20 seconds.

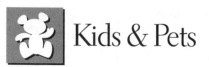

## Kids & Pets

■ To remove pet odors from carpeting, sprinkle baking soda on the smelly area. Let it stand for about half an hour, then vacuum it up.

■ Get your rain-soaked dog smelling sweet again by "powdering" him with baking soda. Rub the soda into his coat with a terry cloth towel, then brush him thoroughly.

■ Sprinkle a generous amount of baking soda in your cat's litter box before you add the litter. It will help control odors. (This trick works equally well in a diaper pail.)

■ Bath time for Fido or Fluffy? Several hours before he takes the plunge, dust him with baking soda to help kill fleas. Just make sure you thoroughly rinse afterwards to get all of the soda out.

■ To make fleas flee from your carpet, sprinkle it with a mixture of baking soda and table salt. Let it sit overnight, then vacuum well. Repeat the procedure two more times on dry days, and you'll be flea-free! If you live in a damp climate, sprinkle in the morning, and vacuum a few hours later.

■ Clean out that old plastic kiddie pool with a solution of 1 gallon of hot water and 4 cups of baking soda.

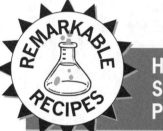

### REMARKABLE RECIPES

## HOMEMADE SCOURING POWDER

Here's a simple cleanser that will get grease and grime off of pots and pans, appliances, tile floors, bathroom fixtures, and just about every other surface in—and outside—your home, sweet home.

**1 cup of baking soda**
**1 cup of borax**
**1 cup of salt**

Combine these ingredients, and then store the mixture in a closed container. Use it as you would any powdered cleanser.

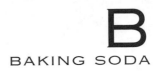

■ To get baby toys clean enough to munch on, wash them in a solution of 4 tablespoons of baking soda and a quart of warm water.

■ Has your young Picasso colored his clothes as well as his paper? Banish the crayon stains by adding a box of baking soda to the wash cycle, along with your regular laundry detergent.

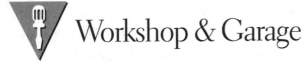 ## Workshop & Garage

▼ To keep your car odor-free, make several baking soda sachets and tuck them under the seats. You can make your own fabric bags for this purpose, or buy them at any craft store.

▼ Clean your garage's cement floor with a solution of baking soda and water. For greasy stains, pour the baking soda straight onto the spot, and scrub it away.

▼ Windshield wipers lose their cleaning power when grease and dirt build up on the rubber blades. So, clean them off periodically with a little baking soda and water on a damp sponge.

▼ Is your car covered with dead bugs and who-knows-what else? Just sprinkle some baking soda on a wet sponge and scrub. (Don't worry—the soda won't do damage to your car's finish or the window glass.)

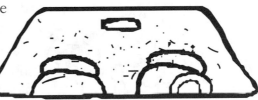

**Jerry's fun facts**

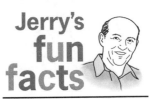

Baking soda is famous as a miracle cleaner, but here's a fact you might not know: Those cleaning powers are severely limited if the soda isn't fresh. So how do you tell if it's still fresh enough to use? Add 1 tablespoon of baking soda to ¼ cup of vinegar. If it fizzes, you're good to go. If it just sits there like a bump on a log, pour it down the drain.

# Yard & Garden

● Sprinkle baking soda lightly on the soil around tomato plants. It will both sweeten the flavor of the fruit and discourage pesky pests.

● Make your own food-safe pesticide for aphids, spider mites, and whiteflies by mixing 1 teaspoon of baking soda and ⅓ cup of cooking oil. Then combine 2 teaspoons of this mixture with 1 cup of water in a hand-held spray bottle, and fire when ready.

● To get rid of weeds and unwanted moss, first, soak the area with a good soapy water solution. Then pour baking soda directly on the plants you want to destroy.

● Clean your outdoor lawn and patio furniture with a solution of 1 gallon of warm water and 2 cups of baking soda.

● For magnificent blooms, give your geraniums (*Pelargonium*), begonias, and hydrangeas an occasional watering with a weak solution of baking soda and water. Any other flowers that prefer alkaline soil will benefit from this treatment, too.

**REMARKABLE RECIPES**

## BYE BYE BLACK SPOT SPRAY

This simple formula works like a charm to head off black spot on roses.

**1 tbsp. of baking soda**
**1 tsp. of dishwashing liquid**
**1 gal. of water**

Mix these ingredients together, pour the solution into a hand-held spray bottle, and spray your roses every three days during the growing season. There'll be no more singin' the black spot blues!

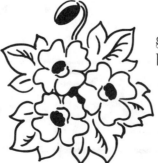

# BANANAS

 ## Health & Beauty

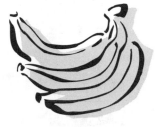

🍎 Here's a facial you'll go bananas for: Purée one banana and one avocado in a blender. Apply the mixture to your skin, and leave it on for at least 20 minutes. Rinse with warm water, and pat dry. If you have dry skin, follow up with a moisturizer.

🍎 Want an even simpler skin treatment? Just mash a banana and add 1 tablespoon of honey to it. Cover your face with the mixture, let it sit for 15 minutes, and rinse with warm water.

🍎 This mixture is just the ticket for dry, frizzy, or damaged hair. Mash half a ripe banana and half a ripe avocado in a bowl. Add 1 tablespoon of extra-virgin olive oil and 3 drops of lemon oil. Mix everything together, and work the mixture into your hair (don't wet your hair first). Cover your hair with a shower cap, wait 60 minutes or so, then shampoo as usual. For badly damaged hair, repeat this treatment up to three times a week until the bounce and shine return.

🍎 Having trouble sleeping through the night? Eat a few bananas during the day. They're rich in potassium, which encourages deep, restful sleep.

🍎 If you have problems with fluid retention (as many women do, from time to time), eat some bananas. The potassium will counterbalance the sodium in your body and help reduce the excess fluids.

 Prevent high blood pressure—or lessen current problems—by eating plenty of bananas. Their potent potassium levels prevent the thickening of your artery walls and also help regulate your body's fluid levels, which are crucial to regulating your blood pressure.

 Remove painful plantar warts with banana peels. At bedtime, tape a piece of banana peel, inner side down, over the wart. Cover the peel with a bandage or a tight sock, and leave it on overnight. Repeat the procedure each night until the wart is gone—it shouldn't take more than two or three treatments.

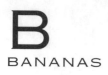

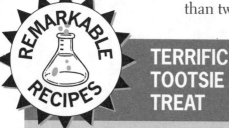

## TERRIFIC TOOTSIE TREAT

Treat your feet to this terrific tonic.

**1 ripe banana**
**2 tbsp. of honey**
**2 tbsp. of margarine**
**1 tbsp. of lemon juice**

Smash the banana. Then add the rest of the ingredients, and mix until creamy. Massage onto clean, dry feet, paying special attention to any cracked, flaky areas. Pull on a pair of cotton socks, and wear them overnight. (This treatment works for dry hands, too!)

# Yard & Garden

● Aphids *hate* bananas. To keep the tiny nogoodniks away from your roses or any other aphid target, just scatter either the fruit or the peels on the soil near the plants.

● To make phosphorus- and potassium-rich fertilizer, let banana peels air-dry until they're crisp. Then crumble them up, and store the pieces at room temperature in a sealed container. When any plant needs a jolt of phosphorus or potassium, work a handful of the crumbles into the soil, and water well.

# BEER

 ## Health & Beauty

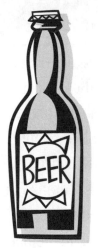

🍎 Make your hair shine and put a little spirit into it this way: Mix 3 cups of beer (any brand will do fine) with 1 cup of warm water, and use the solution as a final rinse after you shampoo. Blot gently with a towel. And don't worry—you won't smell like a brewery. The aroma will disappear as your hair dries.

🍎 Beer also works wonders as a setting lotion. Just pour it into a spray bottle, and spritz your hair before styling it into the "do" of your choice.

🍎 Hops (one of the main ingredients in beer) is an old-time cure for dandruff. To get rid of the flakes, just add a good squirt or two of beer to your regular shampoo.

🍎 After a long, hard day, relax in a beer bath to soothe your spirit and soften your skin. Just pour three bottles of brew into a tub of hot water, settle in, and think lovely thoughts!

🍎 You can drink beer and improve your health! Scientific studies have shown that quaffing one or two beers a day will reduce your likelihood of suffering a stroke, heart problems, or vascular disease.

# B
BEER

Thomas Jefferson, one of our most sociable – and quotable – Founding Fathers, once said, "Beer, if drank (sic) in moderation, softens the temper, cheers the spirit, and promotes health." I'll drink to that, Mr. President!

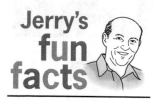

## Yard & Garden

● Your houseplants will have brighter, more vibrant colors if you wash their leaves with a little beer once a week. (Just be sure to rinse them well.)

● To get your geraniums (*Pelargonium*) off to a strong start, apply 1 tablespoon of Epsom salts for each 4 inches of pot size, and water them with a solution of 1 cup of beer, 2 teaspoons of baby shampoo, and ¼ cup of instant tea granules per gallon of water.

● Your clematis will put on a regal show if you feed it from a 2-gallon sprinkling can filled with warm water, 1 cup of beer, 2 tablespoons of Fish Emulsion (available at garden centers), 2 tablespoons of baby shampoo, and 4 tablespoons of ammonia.

● Building a new compost pile? After you've added each 6- to 8-inch layer of organic matter, sprinkle a can of beer over the top. It will launch the break-down process into high gear.

● If it's feeding time for your houseplants and you're fresh out of their usual chow, just give them a drink of beer instead. It's one of the best all-purpose fertilizers a plant could ask for!

● When you transplant roses, ease the transition to their new homes with this terrific tonic: Mix ½ can of beer and 1 tablespoon each of ammonia, instant tea granules, and baby shampoo in 1 gallon of water. Then add 1 cup of the solution to each hole at transplant time.

● You'll have a bumper strawberry harvest if you soak your plants' roots in this elixir before you tuck them into their holes: Mix 1 can of beer, 2 tablespoons of dishwashing liquid, and ¼ cup of cold coffee in 2 gallons of water. Soak the bare roots in the solution for about 10 minutes. Save the solution to dribble on the soil around the berries after planting.

● Want to give your new flowerpots an antique look? Mix ½ can of beer, ½ teaspoon of sugar, and 1 cup of moss on low speed in a blender. Then paint the mixture on the outside of the containers. In a week or so, moss and lichen will start to form.

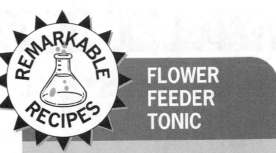

## REMARKABLE RECIPES

## FLOWER FEEDER TONIC

This healthy mix of supermarket super products includes potent doses of all of the "Big Three" plant nutrients (nitrogen, phosphorus, and potassium), plus essential trace minerals. In other words, everything your perennials need to churn out beautiful blossoms year after year.

**1 can of beer**
**2 tbsp. of Fish Emulsion**
**2 tbsp. of dishwashing liquid**
**2 tbsp. of ammonia**
**2 tbsp. of hydrogen peroxide**
**2 tbsp. of whiskey**
**1 tbsp. of clear corn syrup**
**1 tbsp. of unflavored gelatin powder**
**4 tsp. of instant tea granules**
**2 gal. of warm water**

Mix all of the ingredients together, and feed all of your perennials with the solution every two weeks during the growing season.

# B

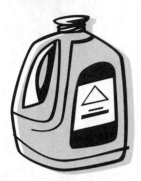

# BLEACH

## Health & Beauty

🍎 For relief of poison ivy pain, pat the rash with a weak solution made of bleach and water.

🍎 Cure athlete's foot by soaking your feet twice a day in a solution of ½ cup of bleach and 1 gallon of water. (Caution: If you have diabetes, check with your doctor before you soak your feet in *anything*!)

## Home Cleaning & Upkeep

◆ Is your coffee mug stained? Soak it for 5 to 10 minutes in a solution of 1 tablespoon of bleach per gallon of water. This method works for tea stains, too.

◆ Get stains off of a non-stick pan this way: Combine 3 tablespoons of oxygen bleach made for delicate fabrics, 1 teaspoon of dishwashing liquid, and 1 cup of water. Pour the mixture into the pan, and simmer until the stains vanish. Then wash the pan, dry it, and coat it lightly with vegetable oil.

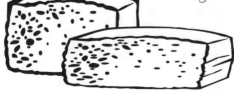

◆ Freshen up old sponges by soaking them for 5 to 10 minutes in a mixture of ¾ cup of bleach per gallon of water. Rinse well.

◆ To clean butcher block cutting boards and tabletops and prevent bacteria from breeding, wash the wood surface with hot, soapy water and rinse clean. Wipe with a solution of 3 tablespoons of bleach per gallon of water. Wait 2 minutes, then rinse.

◆ Clean caulking around bathtubs by scrubbing it with a solution of ¾ cup of bleach per gallon of water.

◆ Here's a good homemade cleaning solution for wooden decks: Fill a bucket with a couple of gallons of hot water, about a quart of bleach, and about ½ cup of powdered laundry detergent. Scrub the deck with a stiff brush (such as a push broom), and then rinse the surface well.

◆ Whiten a porcelain sink by filling it with a solution of ¾ cup of bleach per gallon of water. Let it sit for 5 minutes, and rinse thoroughly.

◆ Clean a toilet bowl by pouring 1 cup of bleach into the bowl. Let it stand for 10 minutes, then brush and flush.

◆ To clean a rubber sink mat, fill the sink with water, add ¼ cup of bleach, and soak the mat for 5 to 10 minutes or so.

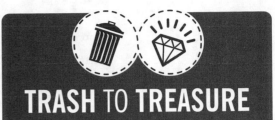

## TRASH TO TREASURE

**WHEN IT** comes to tackling really tough jobs, sturdy 1-gallon bleach jugs win the heavyweight title, hands down. Here are five super ideas for their second careers:

1. **BUOY:** Screw the cap on good and tight, then tie a rope to the handle and a weight to the other end of the rope.

2. **CLOTHESPIN HOLDER:** Cut a hole in the side opposite the handle. Punch small holes in the bottom for drainage, and hang it on the clothesline.

3. **DUMBBELLS:** Pour sand into two bottles until they're heavy enough for your exercise program. When you're ready to handle more weight, simply add more sand.

4. **FUNNEL:** Remove the cap, cut the jug in half, and keep it in the trunk of your car as an emergency funnel for motor oil, antifreeze, or water.

5. **SCOOP:** Cut diagonally across the bottom, screw the top back on, and use it to scoop up sand, fertilizer, compost, cat litter, or just about any other non-edible substance.

◆ Bleach is a whiz at cleaning mildew from shower curtains, shower caddies, bath mats, plastic soap dishes, and other plastic bathroom accessories. Just put everything into the bathtub, fill it with 2 gallons of water, and add 1½ cups of bleach. Let the gear soak for 5 to 10 minutes, then rinse and drain. While you're at it, sponge down the tub because the bleach will clean that, too.

◆ To deodorize your garbage disposal, pour a cup or so of bleach down the drain, and run hot water for a couple of minutes.

◆ Make glasses sparkle and silverware shine by adding a capful of bleach to the dishwasher before a cleaning cycle.

## REMARKABLE RECIPES

## SKUNK ODOR-OUT TONIC

When a skunk comes a-callin' and leaves some fragrant evidence behind, reach for this easy remedy.

**1 cup of bleach or vinegar**
**1 tbsp. of dishwashing liquid**
**2½ gal. of warm water**

Mix all of these ingredients in a bucket and thoroughly saturate walls, stairs, or anything else your local skunk has left his mark on.

*Caution:* Use this tonic only on non-living things—not on pets or humans.

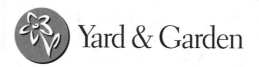

# Yard & Garden

● Before you start any seed or plant in a container that's been used before, soak the pot for at least 15 minutes in a mix of 1 part bleach to 8 parts hot water.

● Before making wreathes or centerpieces from fresh greens, soak the stems overnight in a mixture of ¼ cup of corn syrup and 1 tablespoon of powdered bleach. In the morning, spray them with weatherproofing spray. Let them dry, then make fresh, sharp cuts on the ends before you start creating your masterpieces.

# BORAX

## Home Cleaning & Upkeep

◆ Make your own dishwasher detergent by mixing 2 tablespoons of borax and 2 tablespoons of baking soda per load.

◆ Do you have fine china or glassware that you wash by hand? Make it all sparkle by rinsing it in a sink full of warm water with ½ cup of borax mixed in. Then rinse again in clear water.

◆ Pamper delicate hand washables by soaking them for 10 minutes in a solution of ¼ cup of borax and 1 to 2 tablespoons of mild laundry detergent in a basin of warm water. Rinse in cool water, and air dry inside.

◆ To eliminate garbage-can odors, sprinkle ½ cup of borax in the bottom of the can.

◆ Here's how to make a stubborn toilet-bowl ring vanish: Combine just enough borax and lemon juice to form a paste, and cover the ring. Let it sit for an hour, then scrub with a toilet brush.

◆ Get out stubborn chocolate stains this way: Make a paste of borax and water, rub it into the spot, and let it sit for an hour. Rinse well with warm water, then launder as usual.

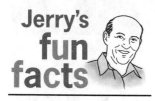

Although most of us tend to think of borax as a common household product, it has plenty of industrial uses, too. For instance, it's used in the manufacture of fire-retardant textiles, photographic developers, and glazes for glass and ceramics. Here's something else you might not know: Most of the world's supply of borax comes from just two places — Mojave, California, and Turkey.

◆ Is there a humidifier in the house? Follow this routine: Once or twice a year, dissolve 1 tablespoon of borax in the water before you fill the machine. This treatment will keep odors at bay.

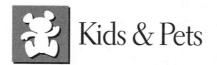

## Kids & Pets

■ Fire departments recommend this method for making children's clothes (or any other fabric) flame-retardant: Mix 9 ounces of borax and 4 ounces of boric acid in 1 gallon of water. Spray the solution onto non-washable fabrics. To treat washable items, launder as usual, then soak them in the solution after the final rinse, and dry. To be on the safe side, repeat the treatment after each washing or dry cleaning.

■ If Fido's fleas have moved into the house, sprinkle borax onto the carpet, then vacuum. (Be sure to get the borax into all of the cracks and crevices in the floor and woodwork.)

■ To get rid of urine odor left by puppies or kittens, dampen the spot with water, and sprinkle it generously with borax. Let it dry, then vacuum the area well. The odor should be gone; if it lingers, repeat a few times as needed.

Yard & Garden

● Preserve cut flowers using a mixture of 1 part borax to 3 parts white cornmeal. Pour about an inch into a pan or bowl. Set your flowers on top, and gently cover them with more of the mixture. Wait three to five weeks, then brush away the covering, and lift out the dried posies. Because the preservative doesn't absorb moisture from the flowers, you can use the same batch again and again. Just store it in an airtight container.

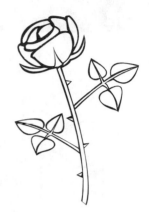

● Beets, turnips, cabbage, and Swiss chard all need boron in their diet. To make sure they get enough, sprinkle borax in and among the rows at planting time.

● If your grass is overrun with creeping Charley or other invasive weeds, nix the growth by applying a mixture of 5 tablespoons of borax per gallon of water early in the spring and again in the fall.

● Got an ant invasion on your hands? Mix equal parts of borax, alum, sugar, and flour with enough water to make a batter. Pour the mixture into shallow containers, and set them in the areas where ants congregate—but only in spots that children or pets can't get to.

**REMARKABLE RECIPES**

## LIME-BE-GONE SOLUTION

This simple recipe will get rid of lime and hard-water deposits on flowerpots, water spigots, or anything else, indoors or out.

**½ cup of borax**
**1 cup of warm water**
**½ cup of white vinegar**

Dissolve the borax in the water, and stir in the vinegar. Sponge the mix onto the lime deposits, let it sit for 10 minutes or so (longer for really stubborn spots), and wipe clean.

# B

# BUTTERMILK

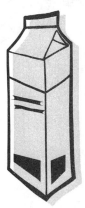

##  Health & Beauty

To tighten up enlarged pores, mix a little buttermilk and table salt into a paste. Apply it to your face, and massage well. Leave it on for about 5 minutes, rinse with warm water, and pat dry.

Here's a great cleanser for oily skin: Combine ½ cup of buttermilk with 2 tablespoons of fennel seeds (found in the spice section of your local supermarket), and heat them in the top portion of a double boiler for 30 minutes. Turn off the heat, and let the mixture steep for 3 hours. Then strain, cool, and pour it into a bottle. Keep it refrigerated between uses.

Troubled by age spots? Make them fade by washing your hands or face in buttermilk twice a day. Or, if you really want to splurge, fill your whole bathtub with buttermilk and have a good soak. (You might want to warm it up a little first.)

To relieve a mild intestinal upset, mix about ⅛ teaspoon of freshly ground pepper in a glass of buttermilk, and drink to your health. (Two or three turns of the peppermill should do the trick.)

## TRASH TO TREASURE

IF YOU'RE like most folks I know, you have quite a collection of 3½-inch computer discs. Here's a great way to corral them *and* get more mileage out of your quart-sized wax-paper buttermilk (and milk) cartons. Just wash and dry the carton, cut off the top and one side, and set in your discs.

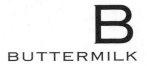

An old Irish cure for a hangover is a tall glass of buttermilk. To cure anything else that's ailing you, heat the buttermilk with a clove of garlic before you drink it.

## Home Cleaning & Upkeep

◆ Wash heirloom quilts and other old textiles this way: First, test the fabric for color-fastness by rubbing a damp white cloth on each different color and print. (Don't just assume that because the red in one print didn't bleed, the red in another one won't— the dyes could be quite different.) Then, fill your washing machine with cold water, and for every gallon of water, add 1 quart of buttermilk (with butterfat content of 1 percent or less) and 1 tablespoon of lemon juice. When the tub is full, stop the machine and gently hand-agitate your treasure. Rinse thoroughly, and hang it up to dry.

◆ To whiten a yellowed bed linen or table linen, soak it for a week or so in buttermilk, and then launder as usual.

◆ Rescue mildewed fabric by soaking it overnight in buttermilk. Follow by washing and drying the material as usual.

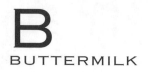

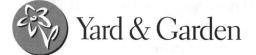

## Yard & Garden

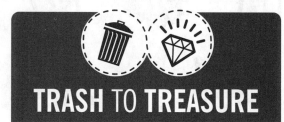

● Here's a trick to make moss grow between stepping stones in a path or on the sides of a planter: Mix ½ quart of buttermilk, 1 teaspoon of corn syrup, and 1 cup of moss in a blender. Dab the mixture onto the ground or the sides of the planter.

● If you already have moss growing where you want it, keep it green and healthy by spraying it lightly with buttermilk several times a year.

● Get rid of spider mites on fruit trees with a buttermilk spray. Mix 5 pounds of white flour, 1 pint of buttermilk, and 25 gallons of water. Keep the potion in a tightly closed garbage can. Stir before use, and spray weekly until the mites are history.

● Are rabbits running rampant in your garden? This old-time trick will send them scurrying. Mix 1 gallon of buttermilk with ½ pound of soot from your chimney or wood stove. Boil it for 20 minutes, pour it into a hand-held spray bottle, and spray your ornamental plants. (Don't use this stuff on anything that you intend to eat.) Stir the mixture now and then to keep it from clogging up the sprayer.

## TRASH TO TREASURE

**IF YOU drink buttermilk and you're growing cabbage-family crops, don't throw those cartons away. Not, that is, before you've rinsed them out and poured the milky liquid on your plants. Why? Because cabbageworms hate buttermilk. Even well-watered down, it'll guard your garden from their malicious munching.**

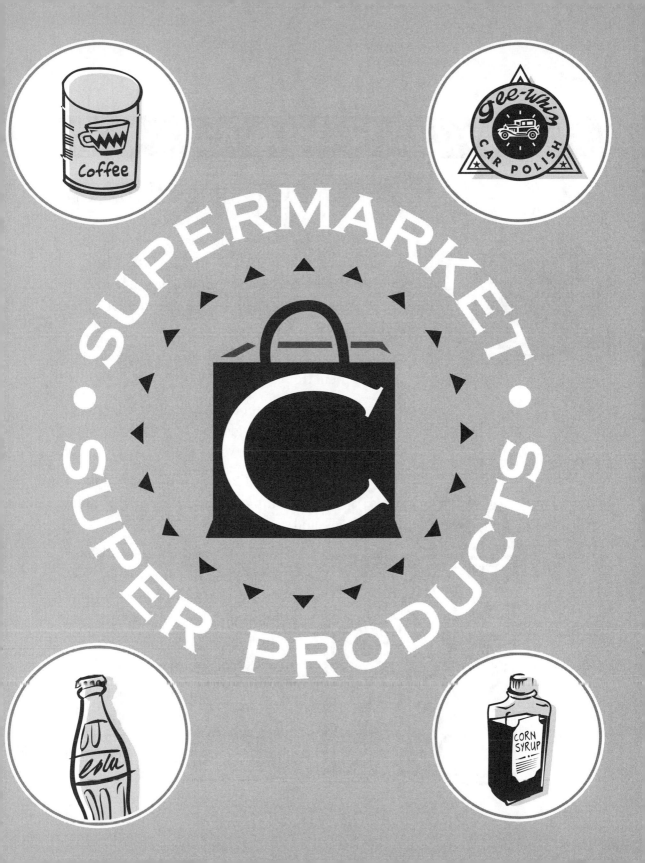

# C

# CAR WAX

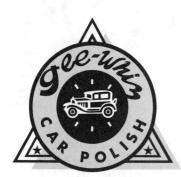

## Home Cleaning & Upkeep

◆ After you clean your bathroom wall tiles, give them a good going over with liquid car wax. The tiles will shine like the sun, and soap scum will have a hard time taking hold, making your cleaning job a whole lot easier the next time.

◆ Rub car wax on drawer runners and window glides to keep them from sticking.

◆ To remove stubborn white rings left on your wood furniture by wet cups or glasses, gently rub the rings with a little car wax.

◆ Car wax is the perfect thing for polishing plastic or Formica® tables and countertops.

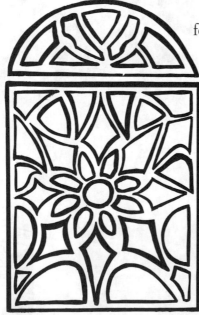

◆ Do you have any leaded or stained glass in your home? Keep the lead around the glass looking beautiful by shining it with light-duty car wax. Just make sure to remove any residue from the glass.

◆ Protect your metal outdoor furniture from the elements by applying a coat of car wax after you clean the furniture. Reapply at the start of each season.

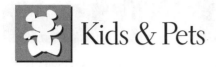 Kids & Pets

■ When it's time to hit the sledding hill, speed up the action by rubbing car wax on the sled's runners or on the bottom of the snow saucer.

■ Got a slide in the kids' play area or at poolside? Make it more slippery by coating the surface with car wax. Give it two coats, buffing in between.

■ Playing cards won't stick together if you rub the backs lightly with a little car wax.

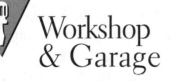 Workshop & Garage

▼ Hey there, model airplane builders—car wax can come in handy for you, too! If you get model cement on the clear plastic pieces of your model, polish it away with a little car wax.

▼ To make bumper stickers easier to remove, stick them on *after* you've applied a thin layer of car wax to the bumper.

▼ When the snow starts to fall, rub car wax onto your snow shovel blade and the snow won't stick.

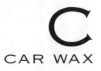

## TRASH TO TREASURE

**CAR WAX isn't the only wax product that's useful to have around the house. Candles come in mighty handy, too— even when they've burned down to mere nubbins. Here are a few ways I use them:**

○ **Lubricate stuck or stubborn zippers by dragging a candle over both sides of the zipper.**

○ **Keep plywood from absorbing moisture. Just rub a candle over all the edges.**

○ **Spruce up clay flowerpots. Wash them, then run a candle around the inside lip to remove any rough edges.**

○ **Give sled runners more go-power by rubbing a candle along the runners.**

○ **Melt them down and make more candles, of course!**

# C

# CASTOR OIL

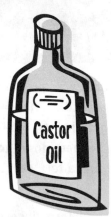

## Health & Beauty

⚫ Massage your fingers and toes with a few drops of castor oil to make your skin smooth and crack-free.

⚫ Soften rough, dry hands with this simple routine: Mix 1 teaspoon of castor oil with 1 drop of lemon or peppermint oil. Massage it into your skin, and sleep with cotton gloves on.

⚫ Get rid of unsightly and bothersome warts on your hands by using castor oil once a day as you would hand cream.

⚫ To erase those little "laugh lines" around your mouth and eyes, dab a little castor oil onto the creases just before bedtime each night.

⚫ Troubled by brown spots on your hands or face? You can lighten them this way: Apply vitamin E to the spots once a day. Then at night, rub on some castor oil. The spots will begin to fade after a few weeks.

⚫ Banish flyaway frizzies with this treatment: Massage warm castor oil onto the ends of your hair. Wait 5 minutes, then wash and condition your hair as usual.

**REMARKABLE RECIPES**

## ALL EYES ARE ON YOU

Here's a great recipe for a gentle and soothing eye-makeup remover.

**1 tbsp. of castor oil**
**1 tbsp. of olive oil**
**2 tsp. of canola oil**

Mix all of the ingredients together. Apply with a tissue or cotton ball to remove eye shadow, eyeliner, or mascara safely and without irritation. Discard any remaining oil mixture.

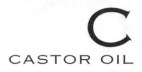

❦ Got a congested chest? Saturate a clean, soft cloth with castor oil, and lay it against your chest. Cover the cloth with plastic wrap, place a hot water bottle on top, and lie down for an hour. Repeat three to four times a week. (And don't forget the plastic wrap—castor oil stains fabric!)

❦ To both strengthen and shine your nails, combine 2 teaspoons of castor oil, 2 teaspoons of salt, and 1 teaspoon of wheat germ. Mix well, and pour into a bottle. Shake well before using, and apply the mixture to your nails with a cotton ball.

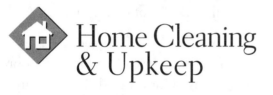 Home Cleaning & Upkeep

◆ Use a drop or two of castor oil to lubricate scissors, tongs, and other kitchen utensils that have moving parts.

◆ Did your favorite shoes get wet and stiffen up? They'll turn soft again if you sponge them off with warm water and then thoroughly rub castor oil into the leather.

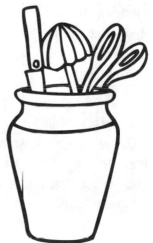

◆ If the wood handles on your knives or other kitchen tools are dry and cracked, rub them with some castor oil to add back moisture and protect the wood.

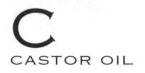

# Yard & Garden

● To rid your lawn of moles, mix 1 cup of castor oil with 3 gallons of water, and use it to drench the mounds. The critters will head for the hills!

● Do you need to protect young trees or shrubs from voles this winter? Just before the first snow flies, mix ½ cup of castor oil and ½ cup of dishwashing liquid in your 20 gallon hose-end sprayer, and saturate the area around all your young woody plants.

● To make sure that your Christmas cactus blooms in December, put 2 tablespoons of castor oil around the roots in October.

● A dose of castor oil will save ailing ferns. Combine 1 tablespoon of castor oil and 1 tablespoon of baby shampoo in 1 quart of warm water, and give each plant ¼ cup of the solution. Your ferns will turn green and fresh almost overnight.

## REMARKABLE RECIPES

### GOPHER-GO TONIC

Got gophers that won't give up? So did I—until I came up with this *amazing* recipe.

**4 tbsp. of castor oil**
**4 tbsp. of dishwashing liquid**
**4 tbsp. of urine**
**½ cup of warm water**
**2 gal. of warm water**

Combine the oil, dishwashing liquid, and urine in ½ cup of warm water, and then stir the solution into 2 gallons of warm water. Pour the mixture over problem areas, and the gophers will go—fast!

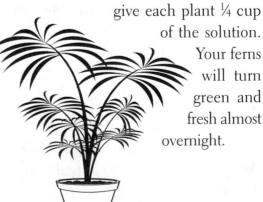

# CAT LITTER

### 🏠 Home Cleaning & Upkeep

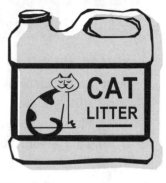

◆ Has your old trunk gotten musty? Chase the odor by taking the trunk outside into the fresh air and sunlight. Then sprinkle clay cat litter (not the clumping kind) on the bottom, and close the lid. Change the litter every few days until the odor has vamoosed.

◆ To freshen up musty smelling books or other small objects, put them inside a bag with a cup or so of cat litter. Check (and change the litter) every few days.

◆ Deodorize a garbage can by covering the bottom with cat litter. It'll absorb smelly grease and liquids.

◆ Going away for a while? Pour cat litter into a flat box, and set it in your bathtub to absorb moisture and prevent mildew from forming.

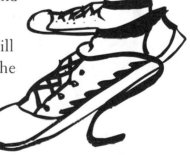

◆ Are your sneakers, um, aromatic? Fill old knee-high hose or thin socks with cat litter, tie the openings, tuck them into the shoes, and leave them in overnight.

◆ Closing up a summer house? Set a shallow, litter-filled box in each room to soak up musty, lingering odors.

◆ Refrigerator smelling stale? Set a box of cat litter on the middle shelf, and close the door. In four or five days, that fridge should smell nice and fresh.

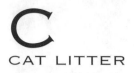

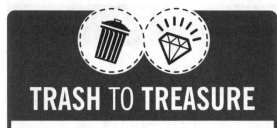

## TRASH TO TREASURE

**YOU WOULDN'T** think that used cat litter could turn into *anybody's* treasure! But if moles are trashing your lawn, Fluffy's cast-offs could be worth a king's ransom to you. When you empty the litter box, just pour the entire contents into the moles' runs. The little rascals will take off for better-smelling territory.

◆ To prevent grease fires in a barbecue grill, cover the bottom of the grill pan with a ¾-inch layer of unscented cat litter.

◆ Treat oily stains on upholstered furniture this way: Grind some unscented, clay cat litter into a rough powder, and pour it onto the stain. Let it sit until the oil is absorbed, then vacuum away.

◆ Make a draft sealer for the bottom of a door by filling an old knee sock with cat litter and stitching the top closed.

# Workshop & Garage

▼ If you live in snow and ice country, keep a bag of clay cat litter in the trunk of your car. When you get stuck, pour the litter under your tires for instant traction.

▼ Sprinkle clay cat litter on ice-covered driveways and sidewalks. It provides traction without harming plants or masonry like salt and other de-icing chemicals can.

▼ To soak up spilled oil or transmission fluid, pour a thick layer of cat litter on the puddle. (The clumping kind absorbs better than the clay type.) Wait 24 hours, and sweep it away with a broom. Scrub the floor clean with a solution of detergent and hot water.

# CHALK

## Home Cleaning & Upkeep

◆ Ring around the collar? Rub white chalk onto the stain, and wash the shirt with your regular detergent.

◆ To remove grease stains from washable fabric, rub the spots with chalk, wait until the grease has been absorbed, and launder as usual.

◆ Clean marble with a damp, soft cotton cloth that's been dipped in powdered chalk. When you're through, clean the surface with clear water to remove the chalk, and dry thoroughly.

◆ To clean and polish metal, sprinkle powdered chalk on a damp cloth, and rub the tarnished piece until it's shiny again.

◆ Prevent silverware from tarnishing by tucking a stick or two of chalk in your silver chest. It will absorb the moisture that causes tarnishing.

◆ Cover spots on suede shoes or clothing by rubbing the marks with chalk of the same color.

◆ Hang bags of chalk (powdered or stick) in closets, basement and bathroom cupboards, and anyplace else where dampness could be a problem.

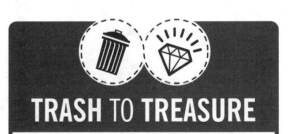

## TRASH TO TREASURE

**WHEN YOU'RE** putting chalk to work around the house, reach for some old pantyhose. They make perfect pouches for holding chalk in either powder or stick form, and they're just the ticket for polishing marble or metal. (For many more uses for pantyhose and stockings, see pages 208–210.)

# C
## CHALK

# Workshop & Garage

▼ To keep your tools rust-free, tuck a few sticks of chalk into your toolbox. They'll attract the moisture that would otherwise cling to the metal.

▼ Prevent a screwdriver from slipping by rubbing a little chalk on the tip.

▼ Got a hole in a plaster wall that's too deep to fill with just spackling compound? Insert a stick of chalk into the hole, cut it off even with the wall, and then spackle over it.

▼ If you've got a balky car or house key, try this: Rub some chalk over the tip and along the teeth of the key. Slide it in and out of the keyhole several times, and you're good to go.

# Yard & Garden

● Say "Keep out!" to slugs by sprinkling powdered chalk around the perimeter of your planting beds. The slimers won't dare cross the line!

● Chalk deters ants, too. Use the powdered version to protect trees, shrubs, and other plants. To keep ants out of the house or shed, just draw a chalk line around exterior door and window frames.

# CLUB SODA

 ## Health & Beauty

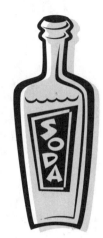

 If swimming in a chlorinated pool has turned your blond hair green, grab a bottle of club soda, and wash those chemicals right out of your hair.

 Hung around in the sun too long? Splash on some club soda to relieve sunburn pain.

 Ease an upset stomach by drinking a tall, cool glass of club soda.

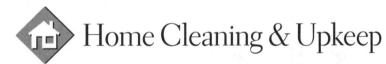 ## Home Cleaning & Upkeep

◆ To clean fresh blood spots, blot them up immediately, then pour on cold club soda. Repeat as often as necessary until the stain is gone for good.

◆ Remove red wine stains with club soda. If the spot is still wet, blot up the excess moisture and saturate the stain with the soda. Rub lightly, and blot dry. Repeat the procedure, if necessary.

◆ Club soda also takes grease stains out of knit fabrics. Just pour on the soda, and scrub gently.

◆ Get your windows sparkling clean by wiping them with club soda on a soft cotton cloth. Dry immediately with a second soft cloth.

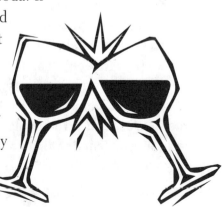

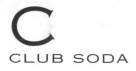
◆ Clean laminated furniture and countertops with club soda. Just spray it on, wipe with a soft cloth, rinse with warm water, and wipe dry.

◆ Soak your gems (both semi-precious and precious stones) in club soda. They'll come out sparkling clean.

◆ Need to get cat urine out of a carpet? Grab a bottle of club soda, and take off the cap. Then stick your finger inside and shake the bottle hard to increase the fizzing action. With your finger still in the bottle, spray the carpet until it's wet, but not soaking. The smell might be worse at first, but don't worry: As the soda dries, it will neutralize the odor—not simply cover it up.

◆ Clean stainless steel counters, appliances, and cookware by rubbing them with club soda.

## TRASH TO TREASURE

**HERE'S ONE** of the best ways I know of to turn those empty, 2-liter plastic club soda (or any soda) bottles into good, clean (and cheap) fun: Make lawn-bowling pins. Just pour a few inches of soil, sand, cat litter, or pebbles into the bottles, and arrange them on the lawn. Knock 'em down with a hard ball of your choice.

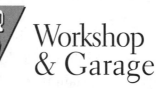

# Workshop & Garage

▼ Clean your car's windshield and the chrome trim with club soda. Just spray it on and wipe with paper towels or old pantyhose.

▼ Club soda removes corrosion from bolts, plumbing pipes, and almost anything else. Saturate a cloth or an old toothbrush with the soda, then wipe or scrub. Let the wet cloth sit on the metal for a minute or so, if needed.

# COFFEE

 ## Health & Beauty

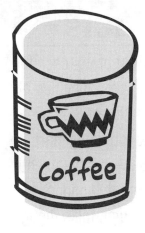

If you're not a regular coffee drinker, and you have trouble with fluid retention now and then, drink a cup—black—from time to time. It's a natural diuretic.

Here's a simple way to put red highlights into your hair, or to cover gray streaks with a reddish tone. After you shampoo and rinse your hair, rinse again using strong black coffee (cooled to a comfortable temperature). Wait 15 minutes, and rinse thoroughly with cool water.

Can't get enough of that java taste? Make coffee-flavored lip gloss. Just put some petroleum jelly into a microwave-safe container and nuke it, checking every 30 seconds, until it's melted. Stir in some finely ground coffee, nuke it again for 30 seconds, and let it cool. Store it in a covered container.

## Home Cleaning & Upkeep

Closets smelling a little musty? Grind up some coffee beans very fine, pour the ground coffee onto a plate, and set it on the top shelf of the closet for a day or two.

## TRASH TO TREASURE

CONCERNED ABOUT cellulite on your body? Rub used coffee grounds on the problem areas. They contain the same active ingredient—caffeine—as most cellulite creams.

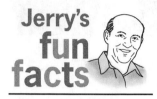

**Jerry's fun facts**

Most of us reach for that morning cup of joe to get the day off to a rousing start. Back in seventeenth-century London, though, folks thought coffee could do more than pep you up. In fact, ads claimed it could cure scurvy, gout, and just about anything else that ailed you.

◆ Keep a plate of ground coffee in your refrigerator to keep it sweet-smelling.

◆ Cover spots on black or dark brown suede by dabbing them with brewed coffee on a sponge.

◆ Dye fabric by soaking it in a solution of instant coffee and water. The more coffee you use, the darker the color will be. Remember, though: The fabric will look lighter when it's dried than it does when it's wet.

◆ To cover scratches in woodwork, mix 1 teaspoon of instant coffee powder in 2 teaspoons of water. Apply the solution with a soft cloth or a cotton ball.

◆ Got a pancake griddle or hamburger grill? To clean it, pour brewed coffee onto the surface (the grill can be cold or warm), and wipe with a soft cloth.

◆ Patch gouges in furniture, wood trim, or paneling with a mixture of instant coffee powder and spackling compound. Just keep mixing in coffee until the compound reaches the right shade of brown. Then fill the holes, and smooth with a damp cloth.

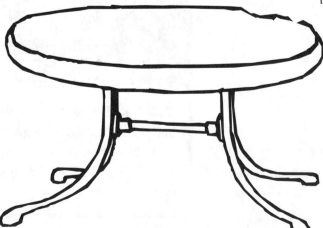

## Yard & Garden

● Water your acid-loving plants like azaleas, rhododendrons, and strawberries with cold coffee.

● The caffeine in coffee increases the potency of any insecticide, so use it instead of plain water in any bug-killing soap spray.

● Pour coffee into puddles and other small bodies of standing water to kill mosquito larvae.

● Add coffee grounds (filters and all) to the holes when you plant acid-loving plants, including blueberries and evergreens.

● When your plants need a nitrogen boost, dig in coffee grounds.

● Add coffee grounds to lower the pH of your soil (that is, make it more acidic).

● To make tiny seeds like those of lettuce and carrots easier to sow, mix them with dried coffee grounds.

● Sprinkle some dried coffee grounds around plants to repel slugs and those nasty cutworms.

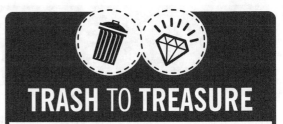

## TRASH TO TREASURE

I FIND it hard to imagine how folks got along before coffee cans came on the scene. Here are just some of the ways you can use these metal marvels:

**START YOUR BARBECUE FIRE:** Take off the bottom of the can, and punch holes in the sides. Then stand the can in the grill, fill it with charcoal briquettes (no need to add smelly fluid), and light. When the coals are glowing, grab the hot can with tongs and set it in a safe place until the next time.

**MAKE REFLECTORS IN CASE OF ROAD-SIDE EMERGENCIES:** Just wrap reflective tape around a few cans, and keep them in the trunk of your car.

**GROW SWEETER MELONS:** Turn a can upside down, push it into the soil until the surface is a few inches off the ground, and set the melon on top. The fruit will be protected from rot and soil-borne pests. Plus, the metal will absorb and hold heat—making the melon ripen faster and taste sweeter.

# C

# COFFEE FILTERS

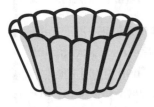

### ◆ Home Cleaning & Upkeep

◆ Protect your fragile china by separating stacked plates with coffee filters.

◆ Use a coffee filter to cover food when you pop it into the microwave.

◆ Keep a coffee filter in each cast-iron skillet to absorb moisture and prevent rust.

◆ Ball up a coffee filter to apply shoe polish or any kind of leather cleaner.

◆ Need to blot a spill fast, but you're out of paper towels? Use coffee filters instead.

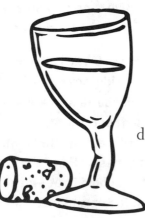

◆ Use coffee filters to catch drips from ice pops and ice cream bars. Just poke a hole in the filter, and insert the stick.

◆ When you open a bottle of wine and part of the cork stays behind, pour the wine through a coffee filter into a clean decanter.

◆ Planning to move? Then wrap glassware and china in coffee filters. When you unpack at your new place, you can still use the filters to brew coffee.

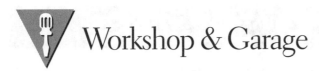

# Workshop & Garage

▼ Clean your car's windows, mirrors, and chrome with coffee filters.

▼ After you clean paint brushes, save the paint thinner: Layer two coffee filters over a clean jar, but don't pull them taut—keep them loose. Pour the old thinner through them into the jar. Cap the jar tightly, and save it to clean your brushes again. (Don't use filtered thinner in paint or varnish, because there will be a little pigment left in it.)

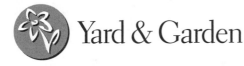

# Yard & Garden

● Cut pieces of coffee filter to put over the drainage holes in pots. The soil won't leak out, and the plants' roots will have plenty of room to grow.

● When you whip up a garden tonic, use a coffee filter to strain out the solid material. Then toss the solids and filter in the compost pile.

● To start seeds that need chilly moisture, put a coffee filter inside a small, zippered plastic bag. Pour 3 tablespoons of water on the filter, and space out your seeds. Put the bag in the fridge until the seeds sprout.

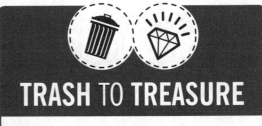

## TRASH TO TREASURE

**DON'T TOSS** your used coffee filters in the trash—toss 'em into the compost pile, grounds and all. The grounds are a great source of high-nitrogen ingredients, i.e., green stuff. One note, though: Once the grounds have been composted, they'll no longer raise the acid level of your soil, because compost generally has a neutral pH.

# C

# COLA

## Health & Beauty

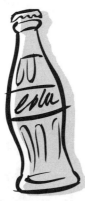

When you take either aspirin or aceta-minophen for aches and pains, wash those tablets down with cola (or coffee) instead of water. Caffeine boosts the effectiveness of both kinds of pain relievers. (So make sure that you don't reach for a glass of caffeine-free cola by mistake!)

When you shampoo your hair, rinse with cola to make it shinier. Follow up with a clear water rinse.

## TRASH TO TREASURE

**WHEN YOU rinse out an empty soda can or bottle—or the glass you drank the soda from—don't pour the water down the drain. Instead, use it to water a plant, indoors or out. Soft drinks are full of health-giving plant nutrients. The same goes for other beverages, including these:**

○ **Beer**   ○ **Juice**   ○ **Tea**   ○ **Wine**

○ **Coffee**   ○ **Milk**   ○ **Whiskey**

## Home Cleaning & Upkeep

◆ To clean a stained toilet bowl, pour a can of cola into it, let it sit for an hour, brush, and flush.

◆ Get rid of grease stains on clothes by adding a can of cola to the regular wash cycle along with your usual laundry detergent.

◆ Cola can keep your kitchen sink clear and free-running. Just pour a can down the drain every week.

◆ Got burned-on food in your favorite pan? Pour a can of cola into the pan, let it sit for an hour or so, and wipe it clean.

## 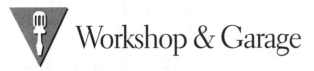 Workshop & Garage

▼ Got a rusted bolt that you can't unscrew? Soak a cloth in cola, lay the cloth on the bolt, and hold it there for a minute or so. It'll loosen right up.

▼ To remove rust spots from your car's chrome, rub them with a crumpled-up piece of aluminum foil dipped in cola.

▼ Clean corroded battery terminals by pouring some cola over them.

▼ Bugs splattered all over your car's windshield? Pour some cola onto an old pair of pantyhose, and wipe the glass clean.

##  Yard & Garden

● Give your compost pile a boost by spraying it once a month with a mixture of 1 can of regular cola, 1 can of beer, and 1 cup of dishwashing liquid in your 20 gallon hose-end sprayer.

# C

## COLA

● Cola is a power lunch for plants because it supplies a jolt of carbon dioxide, which plants need to convert the sun's energy into food. To serve it properly, surround your plants with a 3-inch layer of chunky mulch like bark chips, gravel, or cocoa bean hulls. Then twice a week during the growing season, pour a can of soda right through the mulch. Just make sure it's good and fizzy.

● When it's time to close up your flower beds for the season, cover them with finely mowed grass clippings, and overspray with a mixture of 1 can of regular cola, 1 cup of baby shampoo, ½ cup of ammonia, and 2 tablespoons of instant tea granules in a 20 gallon hose-end sprayer.

● Before you plant your vegetable garden, saturate the soil with the following, mixed in your 20 gallon hose-end sprayer: 1 can of beer; ½ cup each of regular cola, dishwashing liquid, and antiseptic mouthwash; and ¼ teaspoon of instant tea granules. Wait two weeks before you start planting. (This recipe makes enough to cover 100 square feet of garden area.)

● Keep thatch from building up on your lawn with a mix of 1 cup of regular cola, ½ cup of dishwashing liquid, and ¼ cup of ammonia. Make the mix in a 20 gallon hose-end sprayer, filling the balance of the jar with water. Spray your entire lawn once a month in summer.

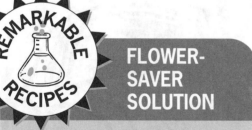

## REMARKABLE RECIPES

## FLOWER-SAVER SOLUTION

Make your cut flowers last longer by filling your vases with this libation, which makes 1 quart of solution.

**1 cup of lemon-lime soda (not diet)**
**¼ tsp. of bleach**
**3 cups of warm water (110°F)**

Mix all of these ingredients together, and pour the solution into a clean vase. It'll keep those posies perky and bright.

# COOKING OIL SPRAY

## Home Cleaning & Upkeep

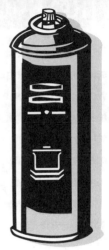

◆ Before you fill a plastic food storage container with tomato sauce or any other tomato-based food, spray the inside with cooking oil. This'll keep the sauce from staining the container.

◆ It's easy to measure sticky things like honey if you first coat the measuring cup with cooking spray. It makes cleanup a breeze, too!

◆ Spray the sides of a pot before you add water to boil. That way, you'll prevent the water from boiling over.

◆ To remove the price tag from an appliance, coat the tag thoroughly with cooking oil spray. Let it sit for 5 minutes or so, and slide the tag off with a plastic scraper.

◆ Make barbecue cleanup a snap: Before you light the coals, coat the grill with cooking oil spray. When the grill is cooled off, wipe it clean.

◆ To get paper unstuck from a wood surface, saturate the paper with cooking oil spray, let it sit for 5 to 10 minutes, and gently peel it off.

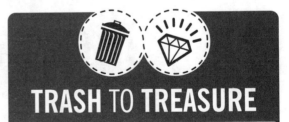

## TRASH TO TREASURE

**EVER WONDER** what to do with those promotional credit cards that show up in your mailbox all of the time? Use them as scrapers. They'll remove wax drippings from furniture or price tags from anything under the sun without scratching the surface.

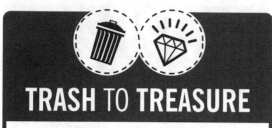

## TRASH TO TREASURE

**COOKING OIL** and all sorts of other sprays come equipped with dandy devices: tall, roomy lids. They're perfect for corralling pint-sized gear like lipstick, mascara, or tweezers in the medicine chest; paperclips and rubber bands in the office; or nuts, bolts, and screws in the workshop. Poke drainage holes in the bottom for mini flower pots.

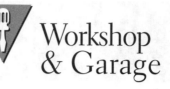

# Workshop & Garage

▼ Got a lot of snow to clear away? Coat your shovel with cooking oil spray. The white stuff won't stick to the shovel, so your load will be lighter.

▼ Lightly spritz all your tools with cooking oil spray to keep them free of rust and corrosion.

▼ Can't get a screw loose? Blast it with cooking oil spray, wait a few minutes to let it penetrate, and your problem should be solved.

# Yard & Garden

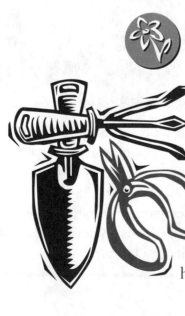

● Save your back with this transplanting tip: Lightly spritz your shovel with cooking oil spray before each use. It'll make digging in the dirt a snap!

● A shot of cooking oil spray will keep grass clippers and pruning shears working smoothly. The same goes for both hand and power lawn mowers—before you head out to groom your lawn, spray away!

# CORNMEAL

 ## Health & Beauty

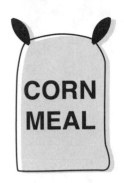

Here's a great way to clean oily skin: Pour a little liquid castile soap into the palm of your hand, and add about 1 teaspoon of cornmeal. Massage it into your face until it lathers, being careful to avoid your eyes. Rinse with warm water, and pat dry.

To get hard-working hands deep-down clean, add a pinch or two of cornmeal to the soap suds when you wash up.

Cornmeal makes an effective dry shampoo. Just work it into your hair with your hands, and brush it out.

 ## Home Cleaning & Upkeep

Got a big, nasty, oily spill on the carpet? Pour cornmeal on it *pronto*. Wait 5 to 15 minutes to let it absorb the oil. Sweep the residue into a dustpan, then vacuum. (You can use cornmeal the same way to remove grease or oil stains from upholstery.)

Here's a simple carpet deodorizer: Just mix 2 cups of cornmeal with 1 cup of borax, and sprinkle the mixture all over your carpet. Let it sit for 1 hour before vacuuming it up.

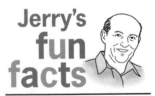

**Jerry's fun facts**

Of 10,000 products sold in a typical supermarket, at least 2,500 use corn in some form during production or processing. So do more than 85 different types of antibiotics.

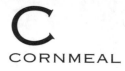

◆ When you get something greasy on your clothes or table linens, sprinkle cornmeal on the spot. When it dries, brush it off, and most of the oil will go with it. As soon as you can, launder the item as usual.

◆ Tackle that tough ring-around-the-collar by pre-treating the stain with cornmeal. Rub it in, and wash the shirt as you normally would.

◆ To clean silk flowers, take them outside, and dust them thoroughly with cornmeal. Then put the flowers, upside down, in a plastic bag, and shake that sack like crazy. The cornmeal will remove the dust and take it to the bottom of the bag. When you're through, empty the dusty cornmeal onto the compost pile.

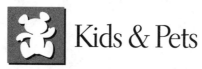

## Kids & Pets

■ Has Fido or Fluffy had a run-in with something oily? Rub cornmeal into his hair, and wait a few minutes to let it absorb the oil. Brush out the cornmeal, and bathe the victim as usual.

■ Clean stuffed animals with cornmeal. Just rub it into the toy, wait 5 minutes or so, and brush it out.

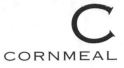

 Yard & Garden

● Preserve cut flowers using a mixture of 3 parts white cornmeal to 1 part borax. Pour about an inch into a pan or bowl. Set your flowers on top, and gently cover them with more of the mixture. Wait three to five weeks, then brush away the covering, and lift out the dried blooms. Because the preservative doesn't absorb moisture from the flowers, you can use the same batch again and again. Just store it in an air-tight container.

● Make your fine feathered friends some homemade treats. Mix cornmeal and birdseed with room-temperature bacon grease until the mixture is doughy. Then add a tablespoon or so of sand or eggshells for grit. Shape the dough into a ball, put it in a mesh onion bag, and hang it from a tree branch.

● Are Colorado potato beetles driving you crazy? Sprinkle cornmeal on the leaves of your plants. When the larvae eat the cornmeal, it swells up inside them, and they burst.

● Sprinkle cornmeal along garden paths to deter slugs and snails.

## REMARKABLE RECIPES

### ANT AMBROSIA

Here's a formula that's lethal to ants, but won't harm kids or pets. (Fido will love it, though, so if you want the stuff to do its duty, keep it out of his reach!)

**4–5 tbsp. of cornmeal**
**3 tbsp. of bacon grease**
**3 tbsp. of baking powder**
**3 pkg. of baker's yeast**

Mix the cornmeal and bacon grease into a paste, then add the baking powder and yeast. Dab the gooey mix on the sides of jar lids, and set them out in your invaded territory. Ants will love it to death!

# C

# CORNSTARCH

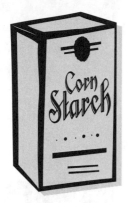

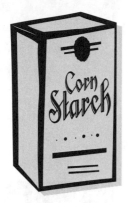 Health & Beauty

 Out of face powder? Use cornstarch instead. But be careful—if you use too much, you'll look like you just stepped out of 1776!

 Want an inexpensive scented powder? Mix a few drops of your favorite perfume or scented oil with cornstarch. If a spicy scent is more your style, add 1 tablespoon of cinnamon to ½ cup of cornstarch.

 Prevent or cure athlete's foot by sprinkling cornstarch on your feet and in your shoes. It'll absorb moisture and reduce friction.

 Are you always getting blisters on your feet, even though your shoes fit fine? It may be that your feet are too sweaty, which often causes blisters. If your socks are frequently soggy, sprinkle a little cornstarch into them before you put them on. Dust some in between your toes, too.

 To relieve either sunburn pain or the itch of poison ivy, add enough water to cornstarch to make a paste, and apply it directly to the affected area.

 Latex gloves will slide on and off easily if you coat the insides with cornstarch.

🍎 Ease the pain of hemorrhoids with this cornstarch enema: Mix 1 tablespoon of cornstarch with enough water to make a paste. Gradually add more water, stirring, until you have a pint of liquid. Boil the mixture for a few minutes, let it cool, and pour it into an enema bag.

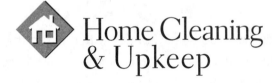

## Home Cleaning & Upkeep

◆ Make your own laundry starch by mixing 1 tablespoon of cornstarch and ½ cup of water in a saucepan over medium heat (don't let it boil). Stir continuously until the mixture is smooth and transparent. Let it cool so that you can pour it into a spray bottle.

◆ To clean really grimy windows, mix a pinch or two of cornstarch with ammonia and water. The cornstarch acts as a mild abrasive. Rinse with clear water.

◆ When you spill something oily on a carpet, pour cornstarch on the stain to absorb the greasy mess. Let it dry, and vacuum up the residue.

◆ Tackle ring-around-the-collar by pre-treating the stains with cornstarch. Just rub it in, and launder as you usually would.

### REMARKABLE RECIPES

### SUPER-SOOTHING BATH MILK

After a long, hard day, treat yourself to a soak in the tub with this mixture.

**2 cups of powdered milk**
**1 cup of cornstarch**
**2 or 3 drops of your favorite scented oil (optional)**

Mix everything in a blender, and store the mixture in an airtight container at room temperature. At bath time, add ½ cup to a tub of hot water, then sit back and enjoy.

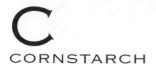

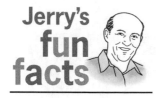

Before the rubber meets the road, it has to meet the molds in the tire factory. And to make sure it slides out smoothly, the production folks sprinkle cornstarch on the molds before they pour in the rubber.

◆ Got a knot that refuses to budge? Sprinkle cornstarch on it—it'll loosen right up.

◆ To send roaches off to that great roach motel in the sky, mix equal parts of cornstarch and plaster of Paris, and sprinkle the mixture behind your appliances and cupboards.

◆ Get your carpet deep-down clean by sprinkling cornstarch over the surface. Wait 30 minutes, and vacuum.

◆ To remove grease or oil stains from smooth fabric, apply cornstarch to the spot, wait 12 hours, brush it off, and launder as usual.

◆ Were you a tad heavy-handed with the furniture polish? Use cornstarch to absorb the excess. Just pour a little cornstarch onto the wood, and rub with a soft, cotton cloth.

◆ When books get damp, fend off mildew by sprinkling cornstarch throughout the pages. Wait several hours until the moisture has been absorbed, and then brush out the starch.

◆ Clean silver with a paste made from some cornstarch and water. Wipe it on with a soft, damp cloth, let it dry, and rub it off with cheesecloth.

◆ If book pages are already mildewed, use the same technique as above—just be sure you brush the cornstarch off outside, so the spores don't invade your house.

◆ Playing cards pick up a lot of oil from the hands they pass through. To get that oily dirt out, drop the deck into a paper bag, add 4 tablespoons of cornstarch, and shake briskly. Remove the cards from the bag, and wipe 'em clean.

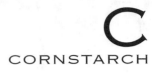
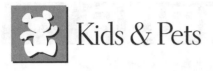 Kids & Pets

■ No time to give Fido a bath? Rub cornstarch into his fur, then brush it out. Presto—a clean, fluffy coat!

■ When you're clipping Fluffy's toenails and you cut one too short, dab the bleeding end with a pinch of cornstarch. It'll speed up coagulation and help ease the pain.

■ Cornstarch will perform that same blood-stopping feat on a bird's foot or beak—for instance, when he's been nipped by a cage mate.

■ Time to change the baby's diapers, and you're all out of baby powder? Use cornstarch instead.

■ Make your budding artist a set of finger paints. Here's how: Mix ¼ cup of cornstarch with 2 cups of cold water and boil, stirring constantly, until the mixture thickens. Pour it into small containers, and add the food coloring of your choice to each one.

■ When the kids want to put on a show, make them some stage makeup. For the plain, white-clown variety, mix 2 tablespoons of cornstarch with 1 tablespoon of solid shortening. To add color, stir in food coloring.

# C

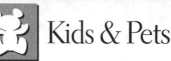

# CORN SYRUP

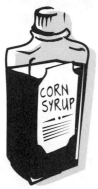

## Kids & Pets

■ To make finger paints that are safe enough for even the tiniest tykes, mix corn syrup with a few drops of food coloring in a plastic container. When your young Rembrandt has finished his masterpiece, let it dry flat for a couple of days, until it's no longer sticky. The picture will have a high-gloss shine to it.

■ Do the youngsters want monster costumes for Halloween? Make some "blood" to liven up the scene. Pour corn syrup into a small container and stir in red food coloring until you have the shade you want. Add a few drops of molasses to thicken the stuff and make it realistically dark. Now that's scary!

## REMARKABLE RECIPES

### HERB BOOSTER TONIC

When the weather turns steamy, even herbs enjoy a cool drink. Quench their thirst with this summertime pick-me-up.

**1 can of beer**
**1 cup of ammonia**
**½ cup of corn syrup**
**½ cup of Murphy's Oil Soap®**

Mix all of these ingredients in your 20 gallon hose-end sprayer, and spray your herbs every six weeks during the growing season.

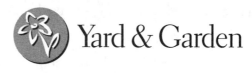

## Yard & Garden

● To get bare-root roses off to a good start before planting, soak them for about half an hour in a clean bucket filled with a mixture of 1 gallon of warm water, 2 tablespoons of clear corn syrup, 1 teaspoon of dishwashing liquid, and 1 teaspoon of ammonia.

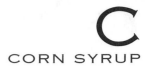

● Putting in a new lawn? First, saturate the soil with 1 cup of Fish Emulsion (a fertilizer available at garden centers), ½ cup of ammonia, ¼ cup of baby shampoo, and ¼ cup of clear corn syrup in your 20 gallon hose-end sprayer. Wait several days before you sow the seeds.

● To extend the life of cut flowers, fill the vase with a solution of 2 tablespoons of clear corn syrup per quart of very warm water.

● In late summer, when your annuals seem on the brink of exhaustion, give them a dose of this pick-me-up: Mix ¼ cup of beer, 1 tablespoon of corn syrup, 1 tablespoon of baby shampoo, and 1 tablespoon of 15-30-15 fertilizer in 1 gallon of water. Then slowly dribble the solution onto the root zones of your plants.

● To make homemade fly-paper, mix 1 cup of corn syrup, 1 tablespoon of brown sugar, and 1 tablespoon of white sugar. Cut strips from a brown paper bag, poke a hole in the top of each strip, and put a string through it. Brush the syrup mixture on your strips, and hang them wherever flies are bugging you.

● Make sticky traps for flying pests by spreading corn syrup on sheets of heavy yellow paper (or cardboard painted yellow).

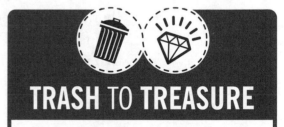

## TRASH TO TREASURE

**PLASTIC BOTTLES,** emptied of their contents, make terrific traps for all kinds of pests. Just coat the bottles with corn syrup or a commercial stick-um like Tanglefoot®. Then either hang them from trees or stick them, upside down, on stakes that you've pounded into the ground among your troubled plants. As for color, most bugs zero in on yellow, but there are exceptions:

○ Apple maggots love red.

○ Tarnished plant bugs, flea beetles, and rose chafers go for white.

○ Thrips make a beeline to blue.

# CUCUMBERS

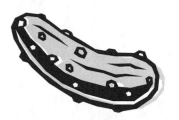

## Health & Beauty

To lighten dark circles under your eyes, cut two cucumber slices, lie down in a comfortable place, and put one slice over each eye for about 10 minutes.

To treat a minor burn, immediately hold the burned area under cold water for several minutes to reduce tissue damage. Then apply cucumber juice to ease the pain and reduce the swelling. (See "Honey & Cucumber Cleanser" on page 152 for directions on how to make cucumber juice.)

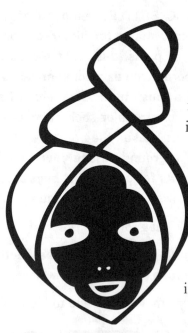

Cucumber juice reduces the inflammation caused by eczema. Just moisten a cotton pad with the juice, and gently dab the trouble spots.

Here's how to make a soothing facial for all skin types: Purée half of a cucumber in a blender. Mix in 1 tablespoon of plain yogurt, apply the mixture to your face, and leave it on for about 30 minutes. Rinse with warm water, and pat dry.

Soothe sunburn pain by soaking in a tepid bath with a few tablespoons of cucumber juice added to it. Or, if you need relief in a hurry, apply the juice directly to your skin.

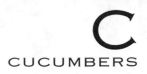

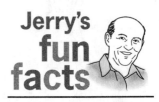

 Do you have trouble with fluid retention? Then eat more cucumbers. They contain a chemical called cucurbocitrin, which helps your blood cells release more water into your kidneys for elimination.

# Yard & Garden

● Got ants wandering where you don't want them to be? Keep them at bay with cukes. Simply cut a cucumber into ¼-inch slices, and scatter them on the ground in the problem area. (This trick works indoors, too. Just put the cuke slices at the ants' entry points, or wherever you want to discourage their presence.)

● Trap cucumber beetles by baiting open coffee cans or milk cartons with (what else?) pieces of cucumber. Check your traps early in the morning, and dump the contents into a bucket of soapy water to kill the beetles.

● Bait mouse traps with bits of cucumber with the skin still on—the pesky rodents love it!

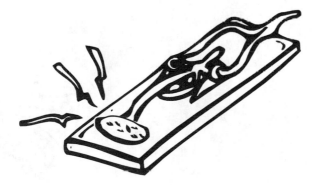

**Jerry's fun facts**

The ancient Egyptians made a fermented drink from cucumbers. First, they cut a hole in the end of a cuke, pushed a small stick through the opening, and stirred it around to break up the pulp. Then they plugged the hole and buried the vegetable in the ground for a few days. When they dug it up, *presto* — cucumber wine! (Don't try this at home, kids!)

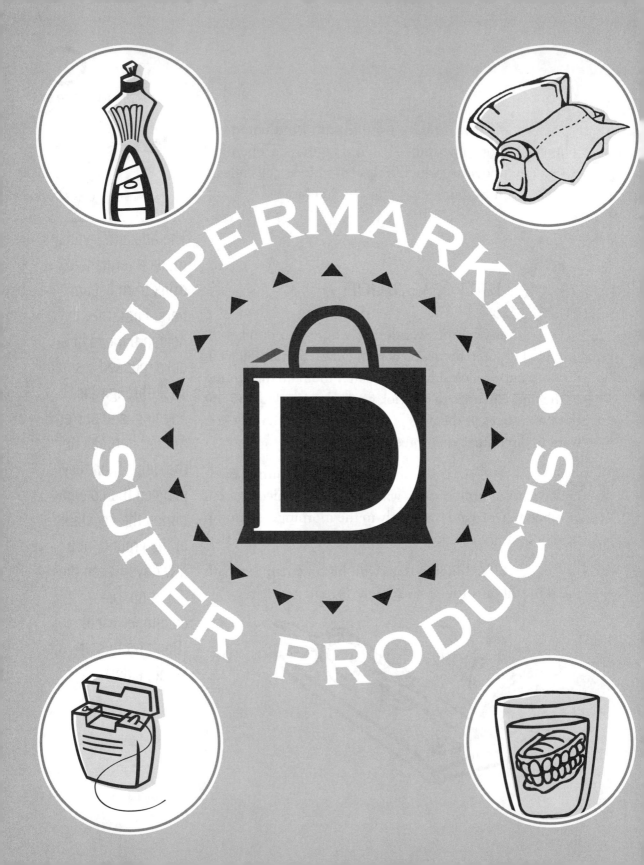

# DENTAL FLOSS

 ## Home Cleaning & Upkeep

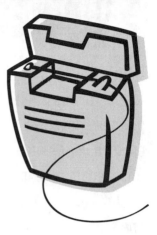

◆ To split a single layer cake into two horizontal halves, stick toothpicks all around the sides of the cake, halfway up from the bottom. Then cut an 18-inch strand of clean, unflavored dental floss, and wrap an end around one finger of each hand. With a clean, continuous motion, slide the floss through the cake, using the toothpicks as guides.

◆ Lift fresh-baked cookies from their baking sheet by sliding a strand of floss between the cookies and the sheet.

◆ Dental floss makes dandy durable thread that's perfect for sewing buttons on heavy coats.

◆ Who needs picture wire? Hang your art collection with dental floss! It's great for hanging sun catchers, wind chimes, and Christmas tree ornaments, too.

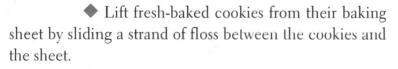

◆ Use clean, unflavored dental floss to cut through all kinds of soft foods, including cheese, cheesecake, and sweet-roll dough. Simply wrap an end of floss around one finger of each hand, hold it taut, and slice through the food.

# D
## DENTAL FLOSS

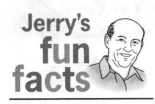
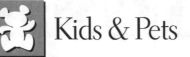 Kids & Pets

■ To repair the mesh screening on playpens, sew up the rip with dental floss.

■ Has the backyard tent got a tear in it? Stitch it closed with dental floss. Use it for repairing other items that take a lot of wear and tear, like backpacks and book bags.

■ Do your young craft artists want to string some beads? Hand them a roll of dental floss. It's thin enough to go through the smallest beads, yet it's much stronger than thread.

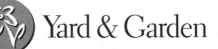 Yard & Garden

● If your sweet pea seedlings are ready for a lightweight trellis and you're fresh out of string, use dental floss instead.

● To make an instant bird feeder, put chunks of suet into mesh produce bags, and hang them from tree limbs with dental floss. Refill the bags as needed.

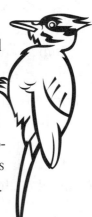

# DENTURE CLEANERS

## Home Cleaning & Upkeep

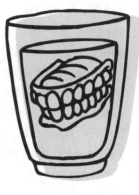

◆ Denture-cleaning tablets are great for cleaning electric coffee and tea makers. Just put a tablet in the filter basket (without the filter), add hot water, and run it through a cycle as you would a normal pot of coffee or tea. Follow up by "brewing" one or two pots of clear water before you make the real thing.

◆ Has your glassware turned dull and foggy from too many trips through the dishwasher? Dissolve several denture-cleaning tablets in a large pan, and soak the pieces until they're sparkling again. Rinse with clear water.

◆ To get your toilet bowl squeaky clean, drop three denture-cleaning tablets into the bowl, wait a minute or two, scrub, and flush.

◆ Sink clogged? Drop several denture-cleaning tablets into the drain, and let it sit overnight. Rinse with cold water in the morning.

◆ Clean a Thermos® bottle by filling it with water and dropping in three denture-cleaning tablets. Let it soak for an hour or two, then rinse thoroughly.

◆ Polish diamonds by soaking them for 2 minutes or so in a glass of water with one denture-cleaning tablet. (Caution: Don't use this trick with pearls or opals.)

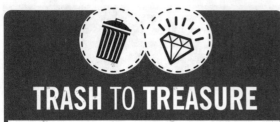

## TRASH TO TREASURE

**SALAD TAKE-OUT containers from the supermarket deli are perfect for storing everything from leftover food to office supplies. There's just one problem: Plastic tends to hang on to odors, and you could wind up living with the aroma of the former contents for a *long* time. The solution: Fill the container with water, and drop in one or two denture-cleaning tablets. Wait about half an hour, and rinse.**

◆ You can remove food stains from clothes and table linens with denture-cleaning tablets. Put the fabric in a container that's large enough to hold the stained portion, fill it with warm water, and drop in two tablets. Leave the material in the solution for the time suggested on the package, then launder it as usual. (Caution: Use denture-cleaning tablets on only color-safe fabrics.)

◆ For a stubborn stain on heirloom linens or other delicate, white (not colored!) fabric, use this technique: Dissolve one denture-cleaning tablet in a cup of lukewarm water, and gently dab the solution on with a cotton swab. Wait a few minutes. If the stain is still there, repeat the process. When the spot has faded, go over the area with a cotton swab dipped in clear water.

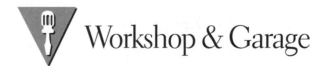

## Workshop & Garage

▼ Denture cleaners work like a charm on your car's chrome. Plop a tablet into a glass of water, and use a cloth to wipe the fizzing solution on the chrome. Rinse with clear water.

▼ Clean grimy car windows with denture-cleaning tablets. Dissolve several in a bucket of water, then apply with a soft cloth.

# DISHWASHING LIQUID

 Health & Beauty

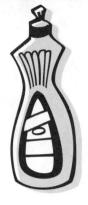

Lather up your hands with dishwashing liquid to remove stuck-on rings and bangles.

Make foaming bath salts by mixing ½ cup of mild dishwashing liquid with 1 tablespoon of vegetable oil and a few drops of food coloring. Pour the mixture over 6 cups of rock salt crystals in a bowl. Stir to coat the crystals, and spread them out on wax paper. When they're dry (in 24 hours or so), put them in a jar. To use, pour ¼ cup of crystals into the tub under warm running water.

Hand-wash delicate lingerie and pantyhose in a sink filled with cool water and a drop or two of dishwashing liquid.

To clean your combs and brushes, mix ¼ cup of dishwashing liquid and ¼ cup of ammonia in 2 cups of water. Let them soak for 5 to 10 minutes, remove them from the solution, and scrape the brushes with the combs and vice versa. Rinse with cool water, and let them dry.

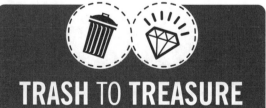

## TRASH TO TREASURE

**AFTER YOU'VE used up all of the dishwashing liquid—or anything else that comes in a plastic squeeze bottle—rinse it well, and set it aside. It'll make a perfect, easy-to-dose dispenser for homemade liquid cleaners, liquid car wax, and many of my garden tonics.**

# D

## 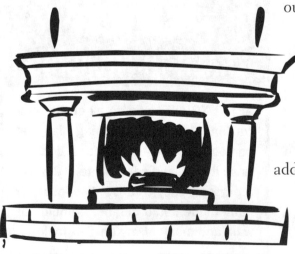 Home Cleaning & Upkeep

◆ Most clothes that are marked "dry-clean only" can be washed in cold water with a few drops of clear dishwashing liquid. (This includes silk, cashmere, angora, chiffon, and even lace.) Gently work the suds through the garment; don't wring, tug, or pull at it. Dry flat on a clean, white towel.

◆ Do you have some vintage, vinyl-covered chairs in the kitchen? Baby them with this treatment: First, wipe them with a soft, damp cloth dipped in baking soda. Follow up by washing them with a mild solution of dishwashing liquid and water. (This formula works great for vinyl car upholstery, too.)

◆ Need to clean the dirty bricks in your fireplace? Combine 1 ounce of dishwashing liquid and 1 ounce of salt with just enough water to make a fairly thick paste. Apply the mixture to the bricks with a soft sponge. Let it stand for 30 minutes, then remove it with a sponge soaked in warm water.

◆ To clean a stone fireplace, add 2 tablespoons of dishwashing liquid to a bucket of water. Sponge the mixture onto the stone, working from the top down. Dry with a soft cloth.

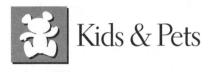 Kids & Pets

■ When your dog or cat has an attack of diarrhea and the semi-solid waste ends up on your carpet, get it out this way: Mix ¼ teaspoon of dishwashing liquid with 1 cup of lukewarm water. Soak a towel in the solution and blot the stain with it. (Don't rub!) Dampen another towel with ammonia, and blot the stain. (Again, don't rub.) Soak a third towel in white vinegar, and blot again. Finally, sponge the spot with cool water.

■ Make super bubble-bath suds—or bubble-blowing solution—by mixing ½ cup of dishwashing liquid and 1 tablespoon of vegetable oil in ½ cup of water. Then, either pour the solution into the tub, or dip in your favorite bubble-blowing tool, and go to it!

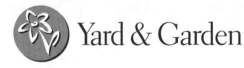 Yard & Garden

● Once a month, give your compost pile a boost by mixing 1 cup of dishwashing liquid, 1 can of beer, and 1 can of regular cola in your 20 gallon hose-end sprayer and applying it generously.

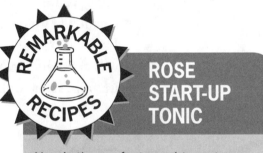

**REMARKABLE RECIPES**

## ROSE START-UP TONIC

Here's the perfect meal to get your bushes off to a bright new beginning.

**1 tbsp. of dishwashing liquid**
**1 tbsp. of hydrogen peroxide**
**1 tsp. of whiskey**
**1 tsp. of Vitamin B₁ Plant Starter**
**½ gal. of warm tea**

Mix all of these ingredients together in a watering can, and pour the liquid all around the root zone of each newly planted (or transplanted) rose bush.

# D

● When you put your vegetable garden to bed for the winter, top it with a thick layer of organic mulch, then give it this nightcap: Mix 1 cup of dishwashing liquid, 1 can of regular cola, and ¼ cup of ammonia in your 20 gallon hose-end sprayer, filling the balance of the jar with warm water. Then spray until the mulch is saturated.

● When you need to go after hard-bodied bugs like beetles and weevils, add 2 teaspoons of alcohol or peppermint oil to the soap-and-water solution below.

● Here's a great way to get cutworms and grubs out of your soil: Mix 3 tablespoons of dishwashing liquid in 1 gallon of water, and pour the solution on the trouble spot. It will bring the lowlifes to the surface, where hungry birds will eat them, or you can scoop them up and drown them in more soapy water.

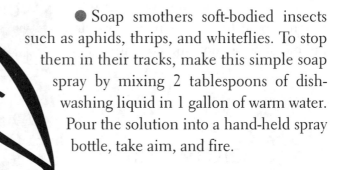

● Soap smothers soft-bodied insects such as aphids, thrips, and whiteflies. To stop them in their tracks, make this simple soap spray by mixing 2 tablespoons of dishwashing liquid in 1 gallon of warm water. Pour the solution into a hand-held spray bottle, take aim, and fire.

# DRYER SHEETS

## Health & Beauty

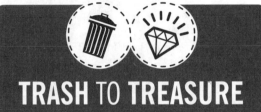

💊 Has dry air left your hair full of static? Get it under control by rubbing a dryer sheet over your hair, from the roots toward the ends.

💊 To keep static from forming on combs and brushes, run a dryer sheet over them every day or so.

💊 Keep a dryer sheet in your purse—that way, you'll always have a pleasant scent on hand without the weight of a heavy perfume bottle.

💊 Headed outdoors during mosquito season? Tie a scented dryer sheet through a belt loop. The hungry rascals will keep their distance.

## Home Cleaning & Upkeep

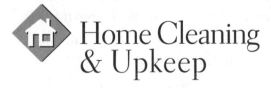

◆ Tuck a dryer sheet into any place where odors collect, such as laundry hampers, diaper pails, or the toes of your shoes to keep them smelling country sweet.

### TRASH TO TREASURE

WHEN YOU take your laundry out of the dryer, whatever you do, don't throw those dryer sheets away! They make some of the best dust cloths you'll ever find—especially for real dust magnets like computer and television screens. Once-used sheets also work as well as brand-new ones for picking up pet hair and lint, and for taking static cling out of pantyhose and other synthetic fabrics.

◆ Line dresser drawers with dryer sheets to keep your clothes smelling fresh.

◆ Between trips, keep a dryer sheet in each of your suitcases. It'll keep that stale, closed-in odor from building up.

◆ Put a dryer sheet in your vacuum cleaner bag. The pleasant scent will spread around the room as you vacuum.

◆ Here's a simple way to freshen and clean the air in any room. Take the cover off each heating vent, spread a dryer sheet over the back of the cover, then replace it in the floor or wall. The sheet will scent the room and help filter out dust, pollen, pet hair, and other airborne particles. When the sheet fills up with "stuff," replace it with a new one.

◆ To get baked-on food off a metal or glass pot, fill it with warm water, toss in a dryer sheet, and let it soak for an hour or so. The crusty spots will wipe right off.

◆ Ready to do some sewing? First, run the thread and needle through a dryer sheet. It will keep the thread from clinging to the fabric, and that will keep it from getting tangled.

◆ Are you plagued by static cling? Run a damp dryer sheet over the offending clothes to de-electrify them.

◆ Are your clothes or uphol-stered furniture covered with pet hair and lint? It'll disappear like magic when you rub the fabric with a dryer sheet.

## REMARKABLE RECIPES

## HOMEMADE DRYER SHEETS

You can make your own dryer sheets and get the same anti-cling power of store-bought kinds, but for a fraction of the cost.

**Liquid fabric softener**
**Washcloth**
**Water**

In a medium-sized mixing bowl, combine 1 part fabric softener and 1 part water. Mix thoroughly. Soak the washcloth in the mix for a minute or two. Wring it out, and use it in your dryer to prevent static cling. You can reuse the washcloth several times before laundering it and starting with a new batch of softener.

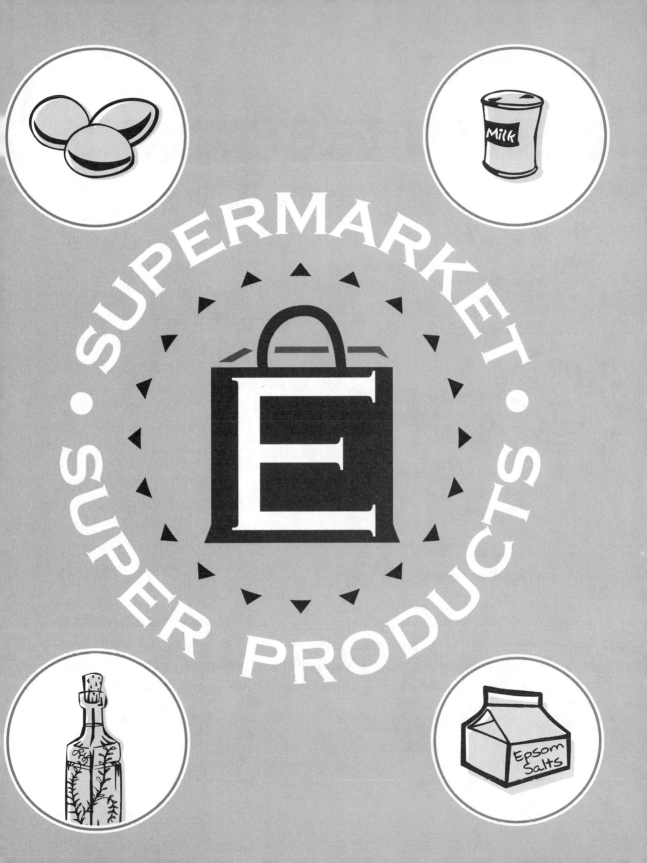

# E

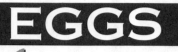

# EGGS

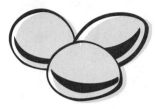

## + Health & Beauty

🍎 Apply egg whites to the lines under your eyes and around your mouth. As it dries, it temporarily tightens up the skin, making the lines less apparent.

🍎 For a simple skin moisturizer, combine 1 egg yolk with ¾ cup of milk. Apply it to your face with your fingertips, using a circular motion. Leave it on for about 5 minutes, then rinse. Store any unused portion in the refrigerator, covered, and use it within a week.

🍎 Here's a delicious recipe for a softening, soothing facial: Thoroughly mix 1 egg yolk with 2 tablespoons of honey and 2 tablespoons of mashed avocado. Apply the mixture to your face, leave it on for 30 minutes, rinse with warm water, and pat dry.

🍎 Got blackheads? Make a paste of egg white, dry oatmeal, and honey. Apply it to your skin, wait 10 minutes or so, rinse with warm water, and pat dry.

🍎 To keep your fingernails looking their best, beat 1 egg yolk in a small bowl. Soak your nails for about 5 minutes, rinse, and buff dry.

---

## REMARKABLE RECIPES

### THICKENING CONDITIONER

This rich blend will leave your hair looking thicker, shinier, and healthier.

**1 egg yolk**
**½ tsp. of olive oil**
**¾ cup of lukewarm water**

Beat the egg yolk until it's thick and light-colored. Then, as you continue beating, slowly drizzle the oil into the egg. Still beating, slowly add the water. Pour the mixture into a plastic container. After shampooing, massage all of the conditioner into your hair. Leave it on for 3 or 4 minutes, and rinse thoroughly.

🍎 Before split ends get out of control, tame your hair with this eggy treatment: Combine 1 teaspoon of honey with 2 tablespoons of garlic oil. Beat in 1 egg yolk. Rub the mixture into your hair, one small section at a time. Cover your hair with a shower cap or a plastic bag, and wait 30 minutes. Rinse thoroughly, then shampoo as usual.

🍎 This simple conditioner will add protein to your hair: Beat 1 egg white until it's foamy, then stir it into 5 tablespoons of plain, natural yogurt. Apply the mixture to one small section of your hair at a time. Leave it in for 15 minutes, and rinse with warm water.

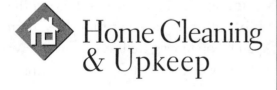

## Home Cleaning & Upkeep

◆ Finally ready to tackle that coffee stain you've been meaning to get out of your apron? Mix an egg yolk with about a tablespoon of lukewarm water, rub the mixture on the spot, and launder as usual. This also gets coffee stains out of carpet—rub the mix into the spot, then rinse with clear water.

## TRASH TO TREASURE

**EGGSHELLS HAVE** more uses than you can shake the Easter Bunny at. This list is only the tip of the iceberg:

○ Scatter crushed shells around plants to deter slugs, cutworms, and other crawling pests.

○ Put dishes of crushed shells in cupboards to repel ants.

○ Soak them in water overnight, then water your plants with the calcium-rich "tea."

○ Start seeds in eggshells. At transplant time, crack the shells and set the whole thing into the soil.

○ Give them to the birds as a source of essential grit. Crumble the shells, and either mix them with the seed in your feeder or serve them as a side dish.

○ Use them to clean bottles and small-necked vases. Grind up the shells, pour them into the vessel, and add water. Then hold your hand over the opening or stick a cork in it, and shake until the dirt vanishes.

# E
## EGGS

## TRASH TO TREASURE

**DON'T TOSS** out those egg cartons—look at what you can do with them!

○ **Separate money at garage sales.**

○ **Store golf balls or Ping-Pong® balls.**

○ **Make an easy, odorless barbecue starter. Just tuck a briquette into each section of a cardboard carton (not plastic or polystyrene!), and light it.**

○ **Hold jewelry and other small items when you're traveling.**

○ **Corral office clutter, such as paper clips, push pins, and tiny sticky pads.**

○ **Store buttons, pins, thread, and other small sewing notions.**

○ **Use the plastic and polystyrene cartons as paint palettes.**

○ **Use the paper cartons as seed-starter pots. At transplant time, cut the sections apart, and put them right into the ground.**

○ **Tear paper cartons into pieces, and toss 'em on the compost pile.**

◆ Clean patent leather shoes, belts, or handbags by rubbing them with unbeaten egg white. Let it dry, and polish with a soft cloth.

◆ Plain egg white makes an effective, nontoxic glue for paper and lightweight fabrics.

## Yard & Garden

● To keep rabbits, gophers, squirrels, and other four-legged pests out of your garden, whip up a batch of this All-Purpose Varmint Repellent: Mix 2 eggs, 2 cloves of garlic, 2 tablespoons of hot chile pepper, 2 tablespoons of ammonia, and 2 cups of water. Let the mixture sit for three or four days, then paint it on fences, trellises, and wherever else unwelcome critters are venturing.

● Here's a simple recipe that will send even deer scurrying. Dissolve 2 well-beaten eggs and 2 teaspoons of beef broth in 1 gallon of water. Let the mixture sit for a few days, or until it smells really potent. Pour it into a hand-held spray bottle, and spray it on your trees and shrubs.

# EPSOM SALTS

 ## Health & Beauty

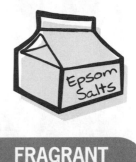

❧ Here's a quick-and-easy formula for basic bath salts: Mix together 1 cup each of Epsom salts, table salt, and baking soda. Store in an airtight container at room temperature. To use, add about 2 tablespoons of the mixture to your bathwater. For a more aromatic bath, add a few drops of your favorite essential oil as the tub fills.

❧ For a slightly fancier version, use 1 cup of Epsom salts, 4 drops of food coloring, and 4 drops of your favorite scented oil. Put into a plastic bag, then shake and knead it to blend the color and scent. Pour the mixture into an airtight jar. At bath time, pour ½ cup into the tub.

❧ Relieve the pain of corns by soaking your feet in a solution of Epsom salts and warm water.

❧ The next time you take a bath, treat your feet to a moisturizing salt rub. Moisten a handful of Epsom salts with a small amount of olive oil. Then scrub your feet until the salts have dissolved and the oil has softened your skin.

## REMARKABLE RECIPES

### FRAGRANT BATH CRYSTALS

Mix up a batch of this beautiful blend and soak your troubles away. While you're at it, make a few more batches to give as presents.

**½ cup of Epsom salts**
**½ cup of sea salt**
**½ cup of fresh lavender, chamomile, or rose buds**
**¼ cup of baking soda**
**15 drops of fragrance oil (any kind you like to match or complement the flowers' fragrance)**
**Food coloring (optional)**

Blend the salts, flowers, and baking soda in a blender or food processor. Let the mixture sit for half an hour or so to dry a little, then add the oil and food coloring. Pour the blend into jars.

# E

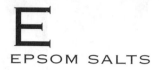

🍎 Muscle aches, spasms, and cramps could signal an electrolyte imbalance. To make things right, soak in a tub of hot water with these additives: 2 cups of Epsom salts, 2 cups of kosher or sea salt, and 2 tablespoons of potassium crystals (available in the health-food section of large supermarkets and in most health-food stores).

🍎 Give your face an extra-thorough cleaning at night by mixing ½ teaspoon of Epsom salts with your regular cleansing cream. Massage it into your skin, and rinse with cold water.

🍎 Use Epsom salts to add volume to your hair. In a pan, mix equal parts of Epsom salts with a high-quality, deep conditioner. Heat the mixture until it's warm, work it through your hair, and leave it on for 20 minutes. Rinse with warm water.

🍎 The next time you have muscle spasms in your back, add 2 cups of Epsom salts to a tub full of hot water, and soak. You'll start to feel the relief almost instantly. Afterwards, lie down with an ice pack on your back.

🍎 If you've got a sports injury—maybe from shooting hoops, showing off on the tennis courts, or returning a wicked volleyball serve—reach for the Epsom salts. Add a 2-pound box to a tub of warm water, and soak those aches and pains away.

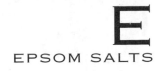
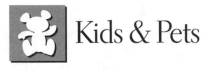

# Kids & Pets

■ When a bee plants its stinger in your dog, first, get the stinger out, then make a solution of Epsom salts and warm water. Soak a clean, soft cloth in the liquid, and apply it to the sting site for 15 to 20 minutes to relieve pain and swelling. If the sting was on your dog's paw, soak the paw in the solution instead.

■ Here's a project that will tickle the junior scientists at your house: Set a sponge into the bottom of a shallow dish. Then boil ½ cup of water, remove it from the heat, add ¼ cup of Epsom salts, and stir until they're dissolved. Pour just enough of the mixture into the bowl to cover the sponge, and put the dish in a sunny place. As the water evaporates, salt crystals will form around the sponge.

■ When Fido pulls a leg muscle, rush him to the vet (of course). When you get home, help ease his pain by soaking his leg in a tub of water with a cup of Epsom salts added. If the pooch won't play that game, soak a soft cotton cloth in the mixture, and apply it to the injured leg as a compress. (Ask your vet how often to apply it and for how long.)

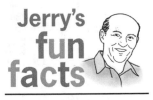

**Jerry's fun facts**

Epsom salts takes its name from its birthplace – Epsom, England, where the needle-shaped crystals were first made from the waters of the town's mineral springs. In scientific circles, Epsom salts goes by the name of magnesium sulfate heptahydrate, or, to be *really* scientific, $MgSO_4 7H_2O$. Besides being a health, beauty, and garden aid, the salts are used in commercial dyeing, in leather tanning, and as a filler in paper and cotton goods.

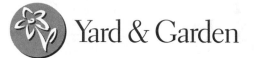 Yard & Garden

● Whenever you feed your lawn, add 3 pounds of Epsom salts and 1 cup of powdered laundry detergent to each bag of dry lawn food (enough to cover 2,500 square feet). Apply the mixture at half the recommended rate with your hand-held broadcast spreader.

● Before you sow grass seeds, soak them in the following mixture: ¼ cup of shampoo, 1 tablespoon of Epsom salts, and 1 gallon of weak tea (use a twice-used bag). Put the container in the refrigerator for at least 24 hours, then spread the seeds out on your driveway to dry before you sow them. The result: almost 100% germination!

● Epsom salts will help peppers and tomatoes develop faster and stronger. To give yours a boost, dissolve 3 tablespoons of Epsom salts in 1 gallon of warm water, and give each plant 1 pint of this mixture just as it begins to bloom.

● In spring and fall, sprinkle Epsom salts around the root zones of flowering shrubs. The magnesium will improve the plants' root structure and the flowers' color and texture. To figure how much you need, measure the circumference of each plant's root zone (usually, the same as the branches'.) Use ¼ cup Epsom salts per 9 inches of circumference.

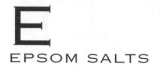

## POLLUTION SOLUTION TONIC

Dust, dirt, and pollution accumulate on your lawn over the winter, causing it to look like a wreck in spring. So, as soon as the last snow melts, mix up a batch of this tonic. (This makes enough for 2,500 square feet of lawn area.)

**50 lb. of pelletized lime**
**50 lb. of pelletized gypsum**
**5 lb. of Epsom salts**

Combine these ingredients, and apply the mixture using a hand-held broadcast spreader. Then wait at least two weeks before applying any fertilizer.

# EVAPORATED MILK

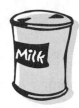

## ⊕ Health & Beauty

🍎 Use evaporated milk straight from the can to remove eye makeup. Just dip a cotton ball into the milk, and gently rub your eyelids. Rinse with cool water.

🍎 To remove full-face makeup, put 1 tablespoon of evaporated milk into a small bowl, and add a few drops of almond oil. Pat the mixture onto your face with a cotton pad, remove it by wiping with a clean pad, and rinse with lukewarm water.

🍎 Here's a simple masque that will nourish and moisten your skin: Puree three or four ripe, medium-sized strawberries in a blender or food processor. In a bowl, mix the puree with 1 tablespoon each of evaporated milk and honey to form a thick paste. (If it's too runny, add a teaspoon or so of cornstarch.) Apply the mixture to your face and neck, leave it on for 10 minutes, and rinse.

🍎 For a super-simple milk bath, just open a can of evaporated milk, and pour it into the tub as the water is running. Rinse thoroughly after your bath.

### REMARKABLE RECIPES

### VIOLET CLEANSING MILK

If you like the sweet, old-time scent of violets, you'll love this cleanser. It's just the ticket for skin that's dry or sensitive.

¼ cup of evaporated milk
¼ cup of whole milk
2 tbsp. of sweet violets, fresh or dried

Put all of the ingredients in the top half of a double boiler, and simmer for about 30 minutes. Don't let the milk boil! Turn off the heat, let the mixture sit for about 2 hours, and strain it into a pretty bottle. Keep it in the refrigerator. To use the cleanser, pat it onto your face with a cotton ball, massage gently with your fingers, and rinse with cool water.

# E

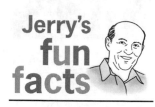

## Jerry's fun facts

A young Swiss immigrant named John Meyenberg produced the world's first unsweetened evaporated milk in Highland, Illinois, in 1885. Canned milk had been on the market for many years, but owed its shelf life to a sugar content of 40 to 45 percent. Herr Meyenberg thought he could produce canned milk without all that sugar. And he did. He called his product "Highland Evaporated Cream." Eventually, it became known as Pet Milk.

## Kids & Pets

■ Do you have a tiny tyke with sensitive skin, or maybe a touch of eczema? This soothing bath is the perfect before-bed treat. Fill the bathtub with warm water, adding 1 tablespoon of honey and 2 tablespoons of evaporated milk as the tub fills. Let the youngster soak and play, and when he or she has had enough, follow with a thorough rinse in clear warm water.

■ When summer rolls around, make sure you're prepared to soothe sunburns and heat rashes. How? Just mix a can of evaporated milk with water, in the proportions listed on the label, and pour the liquid into ice cube trays. Then, when a youngster's skin needs comfort *fast*, pull out a cube, and rub it gently over the trouble spots.

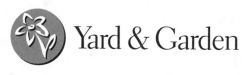

## Yard & Garden

● Protect your plants from viruses by spraying them every few weeks with a solution made of 1 tablespoon of evaporated milk in 1 gallon of water. Use a hand-held sprayer, and be sure to get the undersides as well as the tops of the leaves.

● Anytime you're going to work around diseased plants, mix evaporated milk with water in a bucket, in the proportions listed on the can. When you make a pruning cut on a sickly plant, dip the tool in the milk bath to kill the germs.

# EXTRACTS & OILS

## Health & Beauty

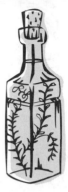

Ease the pain of a minor grease burn by gently dabbing a little vanilla extract onto the trouble spot.

Does the thought of drinking a fizzy antacid remedy make you gag? Disguise the taste by adding a few drops of flavored extract to the mixture.

If you've got dry skin— and not much time to fuss with elaborate cleansing routines—try this simple scrub. Apply a little sesame oil to your face and neck, and scrub gently with a warm, damp washcloth. Rinse with warm water, and pat dry. That's all there is to it!

Rub peanut, avocado, or sesame oil on your face for a nice, natural moisturizer. Leave it on for about 10 minutes, rinse with warm water, and pat dry.

Fresh out of perfume? Put a dab of your favorite extract or sweet-scented oil behind each ear instead. Want some ideas? Try orange, lemon, almond, or vanilla. Any of them will make folks say, "What *is* that wonderful scent you're wearing?"

### REMARKABLE RECIPES

### EASY CALLUS REMOVER

If you use a cane or walker, or know someone who does, then this recipe has your name written all over it. It will gently remove those annoying calluses that develop in the palms of your hands.

**1–2 tbsp. of cornmeal**
**1 tbsp. of avocado oil**

Mix the ingredients together to form a paste with a meal-like texture. Take the mixture in the palm of your hand, and rub both hands together, working the gritty stuff into the calluses and around your fingers. Repeat once or twice a week, and before you know it, your skin will be soft and smooth again.

🍎 Fly-away hair will stay put when you use this conditioning treatment: Combine 2 tablespoons of garlic oil with 1 teaspoon of honey, then beat in one egg. Rub the mixture into your hair, one small section at a time, and cover your hair with a shower cap. Wait 30 minutes, rinse thoroughly, and shampoo as usual.

🍎 Do you go for fresh, minty aromas in a big way? Then here's a bath powder just for you: Combine 5 tablespoons of talcum powder, 1 tablespoon of cornstarch, and 2 drops of peppermint oil in a bowl, and mix well with a wooden spoon. Pour the mixture into a shaker (like a giant salt shaker) or a container with a lid and a big powder puff.

## REMARKABLE RECIPES

### EASY ENERGIZING BATH

When hot, muggy weather lays you flat, or anytime you need a quick pick-me-up, pour this formula into your bathtub.

**½ cup of lime juice**
**½ cup of lemon juice**
**5–6 drops of lemon extract**
**½ cup of baking soda***

Mix the ingredients in a bowl, and pour into tepid bathwater. After soaking in this, you'll be ready for action!

*\* Add only if you have hard water.*

## 🏠 Home Cleaning & Upkeep

◆ Here's a nose-pleasing idea for your whole house: Soak cotton balls in vanilla extract, and tuck them behind the covers in your heat registers. The result is a scent that's subtle, but strong enough to mask unpleasant odors.

◆ To send that "something's baking" aroma wafting from your kitchen, set a dish of vanilla extract in the oven, and turn it on low. Yum!

◆ Make your own furniture polish by mixing 1 cup of mineral oil and 1 teaspoon of lemon oil. Store it in a pump-type spray bottle. To use, shake the bottle well, spray surfaces lightly, and rub the oil into the wood with a soft cloth.

 ## Kids & Pets

■ Keep the family felines from frolicking in your houseplants: Saturate some cotton balls with lemon oil, and set them on top of the soil in the pots. Use one ball for a small- to medium-sized plant, and two or three for big ones.

■ Help keep your dog or cat in the pink of health by adding a little flaxseed oil to his food every day. (You'll find it in the refrigerated health-food section of the supermarket.) It's rich in omega-3 fatty acids, which lower cholesterol and reduce the risk of cancer. Ask your veterinarian to recommend a dosage that's right for your pet's weight.

■ If your child or grandchild falls victim to head lice, don't panic! Just wash the child's hair as usual, adding 2 teaspoons of coconut oil to the regular shampoo (coconut oil is lethal to lice). Lather thoroughly, rinse, and repeat. Wrap the child's head in a towel, and leave it on for half an hour. Remove the towel, and comb the hair with a nit comb. Finally, wash the hair again, and rinse.

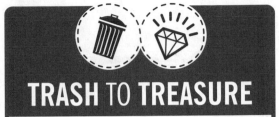

## TRASH TO TREASURE

**MANY FLAVORED** oils come in fancy-shaped, colorful bottles that are almost works of art. So don't even think about throwing them away! When you've used up all of the oil, turn the bottles into bud vases, or use them to hold homemade lotions and potions, herbal vinegars, or even dishwashing liquid. (Just pop in a cork with a pour spout; you can usually find them in housewares stores or the supermarket's kitchen-gadget section.)

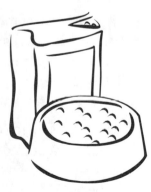

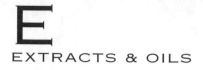

# E

EXTRACTS & OILS

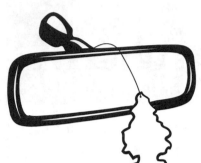

## Workshop & Garage

▼ Make a simply delicious air freshener for your car by soaking a cotton ball in vanilla extract and putting it under the front seat.

▼ To mask unpleasant paint odors, indoors or out, pour 1 ounce of vanilla extract into a 1-gallon can of paint, and mix it in well before using.

### REMARKABLE RECIPES

## ALL-AROUND DISEASE DEFENDER

When cool, damp weather strikes, protect your plants from a variety of fungus diseases with this classic defense mix.

**1 cup of chamomile tea**
**1 tsp. of dishwashing liquid**
**½ tsp. of vegetable oil**
**½ tsp. of peppermint oil**
**1 gal. of warm water**

Mix all of the ingredients in a bucket. Mist-spray your plants thoroughly every week or so when temperatures are below 75°F.

## Yard & Garden

● Need a potent insecticide *right now?* This one will kill some of the peskiest pests around, including aphids, leafhoppers, cabbageworms, and even mosquitoes. Just mix 1 tablespoon of garlic oil and 3 drops of dishwashing liquid in 1 quart of water in a hand-held spray bottle, and spray your troubles away.

● Keep frisky felines and cunning canines out of your flower beds by spraying the perimeters with a mixture of 2 tablespoons of orange or lemon extract per gallon of water, using a hand-held spray bottle. Dogs and cats hate the smell of citrus!

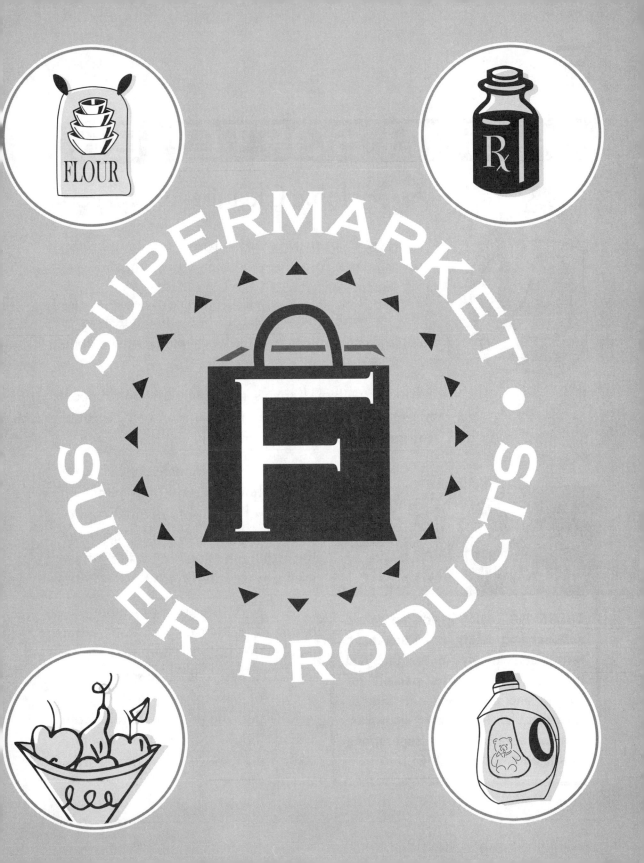

# F

# FABRIC SOFTENER

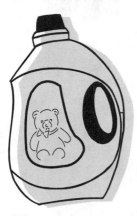

![house icon] Home Cleaning & Upkeep

◆ To make your pantyhose last longer, after you wash them, rinse them in water with a drop or two of fabric softener mixed in.

◆ Use a few drops of fabric softener in a cup of water to clean dust-catchers like glass-topped tables, computer screens, and plastic stereo lids.

◆ Banish soap scum from glass shower doors by using a soft cloth dipped in a solution of 1 capful of fabric softener to 1 quart warm water.

◆ Eliminate static cling on a vinyl shower-curtain liner by mixing 1 capful of fabric softener in 2 cups of water in a spray bottle, and spraying the liner from top to bottom. If the curtain itself is vinyl, spray it, too.

◆ Fresh out of fabric deodorizing spray—or just don't want to pay the price? Then make your own. Mix 2 cups of fabric softener and 2 cups of baking soda in 4 cups of warm water, and pour the solution into a spray bottle. Shake it well before using it to remove odors from carpet and upholstery.

## TRASH TO TREASURE

THOSE BIG, colorful lids on fabric softener and detergent bottles make terrific stacking toys for tiny tots. And the sturdy bottles are perfect for storing and dispensing cat litter or rock salt onto ice-covered sidewalks. (For more ways to reuse superstrong plastic bottles, see page 45.)

◆ Here's a simple way to remove old wallpaper: Mix 1 capful of fabric softener in a bucket with 1 quart of hot water, and sponge the solution onto the wall. Wait 20 minutes, then peel off the paper.

◆ Got a new pair of jeans that feels hard as a rock? Fill your washing machine with water, add 1 capful of fabric softener, and soak the pants overnight. In the morning, run them through the rinse cycle, then pop them in the dryer.

◆ Are your carpets shocking you with static electricity? Mix 1 capful of fabric softener with 2 cups of water in a spray bottle, and lightly spray the rugs.

◆ Give new life to used dryer sheets. Just dip a sheet into a bottle of fabric softener, squeeze the excess back into the container, and toss the sheet into the dryer.

## Workshop & Garage

▼ Clean paint-covered brushes fast by soaking them for 10 seconds in a mixture of ½ cup of liquid fabric softener and 1 gallon of water. They'll come out clean and soft as new.

▼ Remove hard-water spots from your car windows by wiping them with a little fabric softener on a clean cloth. After 10 minutes, rinse with a damp cloth.

# F

# FIRST-AID SUPPLIES

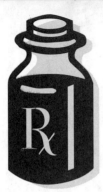

## Health & Beauty

Smooth mentholated rub onto your arms, legs, and neck to repel mosquitoes, ticks, and other bad biting bugs.

Are you battling a nasty toenail fungus? Work mentholated rub into the skin around the nail. Repeat twice a day until the fungus is gone. If you're prone to nail fungi, use mentholated rub daily to prevent outbreaks.

Got a bad headache? Cure it by massaging mentholated rub into your temples and forehead.

When you get a bee sting, the first thing you must do is get that stinger out. Then wet the skin, and rub an aspirin tablet over the stricken site to control inflammation and ease the pain. (This trick works with all kinds of bug bites, too.)

If you have oily skin, the best moisturizing masque you can find is as close as the first-aid aisle at the supermarket. Just apply a thin layer of milk of magnesia to your face, wait about 10 minutes, and rinse with warm water.

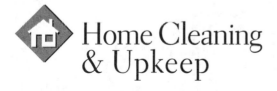

❦ To coax a stubborn splinter to the surface, cover it with an adhesive bandage, and leave it in place overnight. By morning, that sliver should be poking out far enough that you can grab it with tweezers. If it's still under the skin, replace the bandage with a clean one, wait another few hours, and take another peek.

❦ Get rid of a canker sore by coating it with milk of magnesia. Its alkalinity will counteract the acidic conditions in which the canker-producing bacteria thrive.

❦ When you've got a nasty cold and your nasal passages are so blocked you can hardly breathe, reach for this guaranteed relief: Fill a bowl with steaming water, add 2 teaspoons of mentholated rub, and inhale the pungent vapors. Repeat every few hours, and before you know it, you'll be breathing freely again!

# Home Cleaning & Upkeep

◆ To prevent ceramic vases, flowerpots, and other rough pottery from scratching your tabletops, attach three or four self-stick bunion pads to the bottom of each piece.

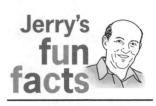

**Jerry's fun facts**

At the 1876 Philadelphia Medical Congress, Sir Joseph Lister presented his theory that airborne germs were responsible for the high postoperative death rate throughout the world. That prompted a young pharmacist, Robert Wood Johnson, to ponder the safety of surgical dressings. By 1890, Robert and his brothers were selling antiseptic dressings throughout the country. The postoperative death rate plummeted, and Johnson & Johnson soared.

◆ Keep wooden floors scratch-free by putting a self-stick bunion pad on the bottom of each chair and table leg.

◆ When your furniture winds up on the casualty list, reach for a bottle of iodine. New iodine will hide scratches in mahogany. For cherry-stained mahogany and cherry wood, use older iodine that's turned a dark brown. To mask scratches in maple, dilute brown iodine with a few drops of denatured alcohol. Use a medicine dropper to drip the liquid into the scratches. It works like a charm!

◆ To keep your white clothes, sheets, and towels bright, dissolve four aspirin tablets in 1 cup of hot water, and add it to the regular warm-water wash cycle. To whiten clothes that are already yellowed, use the same formula, but let them soak for 30 minutes before you hit the start button.

## TRASH TO TREASURE

**WHEN YOU'VE** used up your last adhesive bandage or the last inch of gauze, don't throw away the container that it came in. Instead, save these until holiday time rolls around, and wrap them like tiny presents with scraps of wrapping paper and ribbon, and hang them on the Christmas tree. You'll have one-of-a-kind ornaments for free!

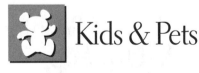 Kids & Pets

■ Do you need a coverlet for a doll-house bed *right now?* Use a gauze pad. To make fluffy pillows, wrap gauze around cotton balls, and fasten it in the back with adhesive tape.

■ When sending a get-well card to a child, be creative. Seal the envelope with colorful, cartoon-character bandages, and tuck a few inside, too.

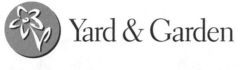 Yard & Garden

● To give your houseplants an extra boost, feed them once a month with a solution of 1 aspirin tablet dissolved in 1 cup of weak tea.

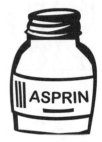

● Need to stake a new tree? Use strips of gauze. It's soft enough for even the most tender bark. Gauze makes great ties for floppy annuals and perennials, too.

● When you mix up garden tonics, strain them through gauze. Pour the liquid into a hand-held sprayer or watering can, and toss the solids—gauze and all—onto the compost pile.

● Are ants invading your garbage cans or plastic compost bin? Smear a line of mentholated rub around the can or bin at ground level. The ants won't cross the line.

● Make cut flowers last longer by adding two aspirin tablets for each quart of water in the vase.

# F

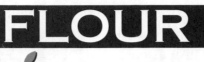

# FLOUR

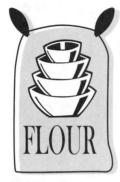

## 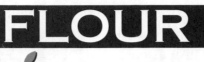 Health & Beauty

No time to wash your hair? Sprinkle on a little flour, then brush it through your hair. It'll absorb any oil and dandruff.

If you've got frizzy, fly-away hair, try this simple cure: Combine 1 cup of flour with ⅔ cup of cold water, and mix until it's free of lumps. Apply the paste to your hair, smoothing the hair straight back. Wait 20 minutes, rinse thoroughly, and wash your hair with a mild shampoo, rinsing with cool water.

## Home Cleaning & Upkeep

◆ Clean chrome by sprinkling a little white flour on a dry rag and polishing in a circular motion. The chrome will shine up perfectly—with no scratches!

◆ To clean white leather or suede, simply rub white flour into it, and brush off the excess. For stubborn stains on leather, rub with a paste of flour and water.

## TRASH TO TREASURE

THE NEXT time you empty a spice jar that has a perforated plastic liner under the lid, give it new life as a flour dispenser. It's perfect for sprinkling just the right amount of flour when you want to polish chrome, clean leather, or perform other non-culinary chores.

◆ Make your own brass and copper polish by mixing 1 tablespoon of flour, 1 tablespoon of salt, and 1 tablespoon of white vinegar into a thick paste. Apply a thick layer to a damp sponge, and gently wipe the metal. Let the polish dry for about an hour, rinse with warm water, and buff with a clean, soft cloth.

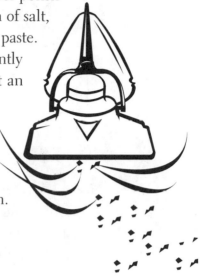

◆ Soak up grease or oil spills by pouring flour on the spots. Let it sit until the mess has been absorbed, then vacuum. Repeat the process, if necessary.

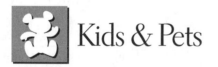 ## Kids & Pets

■ Make a kid-safe (and furniture-safe) paste by mixing flour and water to a pancake-batter consistency. This adhesive works like a charm on paper, lightweight fabric, and cardboard.

■ Make modeling clay this way: In a saucepan, mix 2 cups of flour, 4 tablespoons of cream of tartar, 2 tablespoons of vegetable oil, 1 cup of salt, a few drops of food coloring, and 2 cups of water. Stir over medium heat for 3 to 5 minutes, or until the mixture forms a ball. When it's cooled, mix it with your hands, and store it in an airtight container.

# F

FLOUR

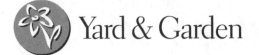 Yard & Garden

● Not sure what kind of critters are munching on your plants? Sprinkle flour on the ground. The next time the culprits come around, they'll leave their footprints behind. If you don't recognize them on sight, get out your Audubon Field Guide to make a positive I.D.

● Here's a simple way to get rid of cabbage-worms and deter other pests: Mix 1 cup of flour and 2 tablespoons of cayenne pepper, and sprinkle the mixture on all your cabbage-family plants. The flour swells up inside the worms and bursts their insides, while the hot pepper keeps other bugs away.

● Dust flour and a pinch or two of black pepper onto the soil around your perennials to keep whiteflies and other garden thugs away.

● Repel ants by pouring a line of flour around their target. They won't cross the line.

● Mice driving you crazy? Mix equal parts of flour and plaster of Paris, and spoon the powder into shallow containers. Add a pinch or two of cookie crumbs or chocolate drink mix to each one, and stir it in. Then set out the bait where only mice can get to it (not children or pets), and put a saucer of water nearby.

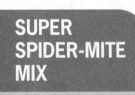

## SUPER SPIDER-MITE MIX

When tiny spider mites are causing big mischief in your garden, reach for this recipe.

**4 cups of wheat flour**
**½ cup of buttermilk**
**5 gal. of water**

Mix all of these ingredients together, pour the mixture into a hand-held spray bottle, and mist-spray your plants to the point of run-off.

# FOOD COLORING

## 🏠 Home Cleaning & Upkeep

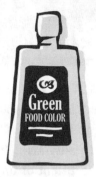

◆ Are you wallpapering a room? Add a few drops of food coloring to the paste so you can see how well you're covering the paper.

◆ To re-color small bleached spots on clothing, mix food coloring with water to make the proper shade, and dab it onto the spots.

## 🐨 Kids & Pets

■ For a fast, easy, and inexpensive bathtime treat, just add a few drops of food coloring to a child's bath water.

■ Put a teaspoon of food coloring in a spray or squeeze bottle filled with water, and let kids have a ball by spraying designs in the snow.

■ Fill a squeeze bottle with white, water-based glue, then tint the glue with a few drops of food coloring. The kids can make raised designs on paper.

■ Use food coloring to tint wooden toys (details on page 122, bottom). Coat with clear lacquer to lock in the color.

### REMARKABLE RECIPES

### FUN & FANCY SOAP

Both kids and grownups love this colorful, easy-to-make soap.

**1 bar of floating bath soap (such as Ivory®), grated**
**4–6 drops of food coloring**
**2–3 drops of scented oil**
**¼ cup of warm water**

Mix all of the ingredients in a bowl until stiff. Remove from the bowl, and knead to the consistency of very thick dough. Spoon into plastic molds or cookie cutters, and set in the freezer for 10 minutes. Pop the soaps out of the molds, and let them dry until hard.

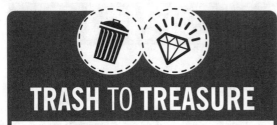

## TRASH TO TREASURE

**WANT TO fill the kids' (or even grown-ups') Easter baskets with the fanciest eggs in town? All you need are some old pantyhose, food coloring, and an assortment of tiny leaves or flowers—and hard-boiled eggs, of course! First, make your egg dye following the directions on the food-coloring package. Press a leaf or flower flat against an egg, wrap a piece of pantyhose around it, and tie it tight with string. Dip the egg into the dye, keep it there until it reaches the color intensity you want, and then pull it out. Let the egg dry inside the pantyhose, cut away the fabric, and *voilà!*—a one-of-a-kind egg designed by you!**

■ Use some food coloring to make finger paints for your junior artist. Mix ¼ cup of cornstarch with 2 cups of cold water, and boil, stirring constantly, until the mixture thickens. Pour it into small containers, and add a different food coloring to each one.

■ Have your teenagers been "dyeing" for a new (and outlandish) hair color? Or maybe you want a drop-dead tint to go with a Halloween costume. Food coloring will do a safe—and temporary—job. Dilute it until you like the shade, and apply it to your hair. Leave it on until it's reached the desired color intensity, then rinse with cool water.

 Yard & Garden

● Tint some white or pale-colored cut flowers by mixing food coloring in warm water and placing the freshly cut stems in the solution. Let them sit overnight and by morning, they will be sporting multi-toned designs.

● Food coloring makes a great stain for wooden planters or any unfinished wood (white pine works best). Mix 1 part food coloring to 5 or 6 parts water. Saturate the wood surface, wait about 5 minutes, and wipe with a soft cloth. Let dry overnight, then wipe again.

# FRUIT & FRUIT JUICE

## Health & Beauty

If you've got dark circles under your eyes, and you *do* care a feather *and* a fig about it, treat yourself to this routine: Cut a fresh fig in half. Lie down in a comfortable place, and put one fig half over each eye for about 10 minutes.

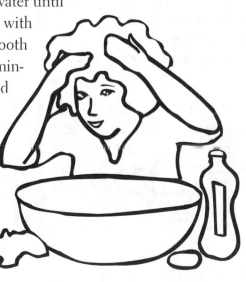

Papaya is a fabulous remedy for dry, flaky, or rough skin—especially when it's the result of a fading suntan. Just mash the fruit, and apply it in a thin layer to your face, neck, and chest. Wait 10 to 20 minutes, then rinse with cool water, and pat dry.

Here's a simple way to nourish and soften your skin: Soak 1 cup of dried apricots in water until they're soft. Purée them in a blender with 2 tablespoons of powdered milk, and smooth the mixture onto your face. Wait about 15 minutes, wipe it off with a damp washcloth, and rinse with warm water.

Want to put blonde highlights in your hair—without the beauty salon price tag? Stir 3 tablespoons of chopped rhubarb into 3 cups of hot water. Simmer for 10 minutes, strain, and cool. Use the solution as a rinse after each shampoo.

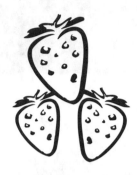

🍎 Fresh out of toothpaste? Just mash 3 large strawberries, and use them as you would any toothpaste. Rinse well to get out any little seeds from between your teeth and gums.

🍎 Troubled by cellulite? Try this copycat version of those herbal wraps the fancy spas use: Mix ½ cup of grapefruit juice, 1 cup of corn oil, and 2 teaspoons of dried thyme. Massage the mixture into your thighs, hips, and buttocks, and cover the area with plastic wrap. Hold a heating pad over each body section for 5 minutes.

🍎 Tired tootsies? Try this fruity nighttime treat. Mix 8 strawberries, 2 tablespoons of olive oil, and 1 teaspoon of sea salt or kosher salt together. Massage the paste into your feet, rinse it off, and pat dry.

## REMARKABLE RECIPES

### TUTTI-FRUTTI FACIAL

If you like the aroma of fresh fruit salad, you'll love this super softening and invigorating facial.

**6 strawberries**
**½ of an apple**
**½ of a pear**
**1 oz. of orange juice**
**Honey**

Purée the fruits with the orange juice in a blender. Apply a thin layer of honey to your face, then apply the fruit mixture. Leave it on your skin for at least 30 minutes, rinse with warm water, and pat dry.

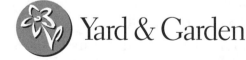

## Yard & Garden

● If you water your plants with tap water that has a lot of dissolved minerals in it, or if you mist-spray your plants with fertilizer, the leaves can start to look dull and drab. What to do? Wipe pineapple juice or any citrus juice onto the leaves with a clean, soft cotton cloth. They'll shine right up.

● Nothing draws rose chafers faster than the ultrasweet smell of decaying fruit. If these beetles are plaguing your plants, fill some jars about halfway with soapy water, drop in some chunks of over-the-hill fruit (any kind will do), and set the jars under your rose bushes.

● Trap Japanese beetles with grape juice. Just set a pan of soapy water on the ground about 25 feet from a plant you want to protect. In the center of the pan, stand a can or jar with an inch or so of grape juice in it. Cover the top of the can with a piece of window screening. The beetles will make a beeline for the juice, fall into the water, and drown.

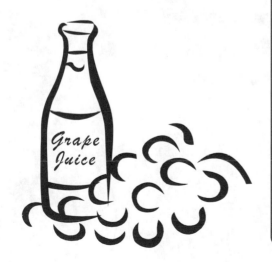

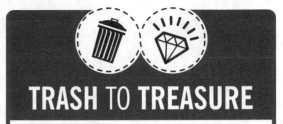

# TRASH TO TREASURE

**HERE'S FIVE fantastic uses for plastic berry baskets:**

**1. EASTER BASKET:** Deck it out with ribbons, fill it with cellophane "grass," and add a handle if you like.

**2. TOOLBENCH OR DESK ORGANIZER:** Turn it upside down, and fill the grid with skinny gear like pencils and pens, screwdrivers, files, or small paintbrushes.

**3. SHOWER CADDY:** Get two small suction-cup hooks, stick them to the wall, and hang the basket from them. Then tuck in soaps, bath beads, your razor, and other personal items.

**4. DISHWASHER BASKET:** Perfect for organizing little things that tend to slide around, such as small lids and tiny spoons. (Use it only in the top rack, though.)

**5. FLOPPY DISC HOLDER:** A berry basket will hold plenty of 3½-inch discs for your computer.

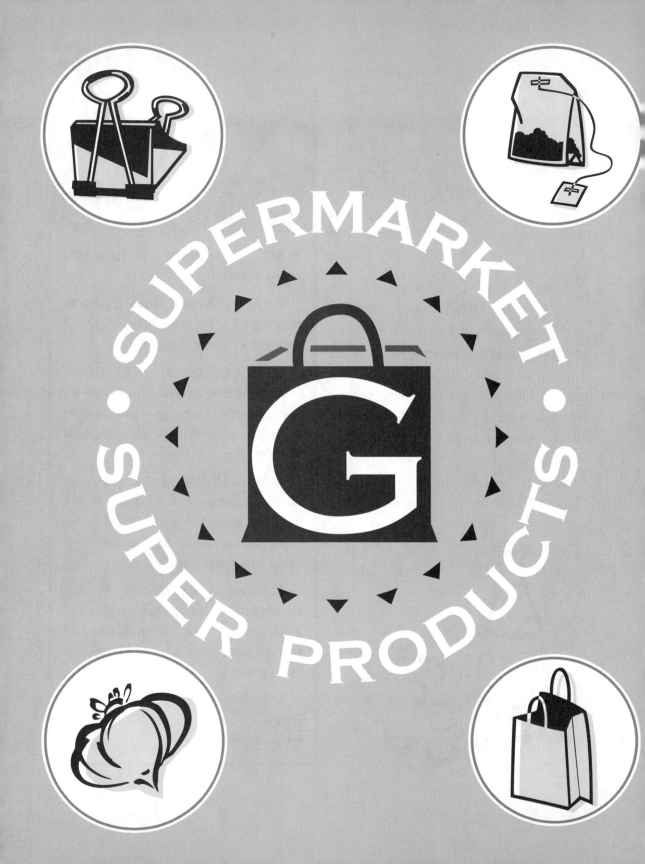

SUPERMARKET · SUPER PRODUCTS ·

G

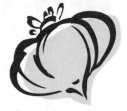

# GARLIC

 ## Health & Beauty

To make blemishes vanish, peel and mash 6 cloves of garlic, and apply to the affected areas (avoiding your eyes). Leave it in place for about 10 minutes, rinse with warm water, and pat dry.

Keep this old-time remedy on hand during cold and flu season to take when needed: Peel and mince 6 large cloves of garlic, put them in a jar, cover them with olive oil, and put the lid on the jar. Let the mixture sit in the refrigerator for three days, stirring every day. Strain it through cheesecloth into another clean jar. Take 1 teaspoon per hour until your symptoms vanish.

Here's a sweet variation on that: Peel and chop a bulb of garlic, cover with 1 tablespoon of honey, and bake until the juice oozes from it. Take 1 teaspoon per hour.

When congestion is backing up into your ears, try this potent (some would say "desperate") treatment. Spread ½ teaspoon of horseradish or mustard on 3 or 4 slices of raw garlic. Then eat this, washing the concoction down with a cup of peppermint tea.

Here's a simple cure for athlete's foot: Crush several garlic cloves, and drop them into a tub of warm water with a little rubbing alcohol added. Soak your feet in the water for about 10 minutes, once a day. (Caution: If you have diabetes, check with your doctor first.)

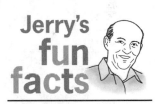

**Jerry's fun facts**

First Lady Eleanor Roosevelt ate three chocolate-covered garlic balls every morning because her doctor told her it would improve her memory.

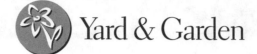

# Yard & Garden

● To fight soil-borne fungi, combine four crushed garlic bulbs and ½ cup of baking soda in 1 gallon of water in a pot. Bring the water to a boil. Turn off the heat, and let it cool to room temperature. Strain the liquid into a watering can, and soak the ground around fungus-prone plants. Go *very* slowly so that the liquid goes deep into the ground. Then gently work the strained-out garlic into the soil.

● Keep neighborhood dogs and cats off of your lawn with this simple solution: Grind up two or three cloves of garlic and three or four hot peppers in a blender. Mix them with a bucket of water and a few drops of dishwashing liquid. Dribble the elixir around the edges of your lawn and sidewalk. Repeat frequently, especially after each rain.

● Tuck some garlic bulbs into the soil among your roses. When the roses come up, the garlic will deter cane borers, aphids, rose chafers, and Japanese beetles.

● To kill just about any kind of insect pest, mix 3 tablespoons of garlic oil (see the recipe at left) with three drops of dishwashing liquid in 1 quart of water. Pour the solution into a hand-held spray bottle, take aim, and fire away!

## REMARKABLE RECIPES

### GARLIC OIL

Mix up this concentrate, and reach for it whenever you need to solve big-time bug problems.

**1 whole bulb of garlic, minced**
**1 cup of vegetable oil**

Mix the garlic and oil together in a glass jar with a tight lid. Put the mixture in the refrigerator to steep for a day or two, then test it for "doneness." If your eyes don't water when you open the lid, add another half-bulb of minced garlic, and wait another day. Strain out the solids, and pour the oil into a fresh jar. Keep it in the fridge until you're ready to use it. Dilute it as indicated in any recipe that calls for garlic oil.

# GELATIN

## Health & Beauty

For a great hair gel, simply mix unflavored gelatin with half as much water as the instructions on the package specify. It'll let you sculpt your hair into just about any style you can imagine.

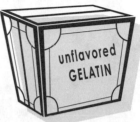
unflavored GELATIN

Here's an easy, peel-off facial masque. Mix 1½ tablespoons of unflavored gelatin and ½ cup of fruit juice in a microwave-safe container, and nuke it until the gelatin is completely dissolved. Set the container in the refrigerator until it's almost set (about 25 minutes). Spread it on your face, let it dry, and peel it off. Great juice choices: lemon, grapefruit, or tomato for oily skin; apple, raspberry, or pear for normal to dry skin.

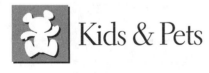

## Kids & Pets

Here's a science project the kids are sure to love: Have them grow seeds in clear gelatin. They'll be able to watch as the root structures develop.

### REMARKABLE RECIPES

### GEL AIR FRESHENER

If you like scented air fresheners, you'll love this easy recipe.

**2 cups of distilled water**
**4 cups of unflavored gelatin**
**10–20 drops of fragrance oil**
**Food coloring (optional)**

Heat 1 cup of the water almost to boiling, then add the gelatin and stir until it's dissolved. Remove from the heat and add the remaining cup of water, the fragrance, and food coloring. Pour the mixture into clean jars, and let them sit at room temperature until they've fully gelled. (They'll set faster in the refrigerator, but will share their scent with your food.)

■ Help the kids make stickers—or make some for the grandkids to keep at your house. First, cut pictures from gift wrap, magazines, or junk mail. Mix 2 teaspoons of flavored gelatin with 5 teaspoons of boiling water. With a small brush, paint a thin coat of the solution onto the back of each cutout. Let them dry, then store them in a covered box until the kids are ready to lick and stick.

## REMARKABLE RECIPES

### CONTAINER PLANT TONIC

To water your outdoor container plants, make this marvelous master mix of fortified water.

**1 tbsp. of 15-30-15 fertilizer**
**½ tsp. of gelatin**
**½ tsp. of dishwashing liquid**
**½ tsp. of corn syrup**
**½ tsp. of whiskey**
**¼ tsp. of instant tea granules**
**Water**

Mix the first six ingredients in a 1-gallon milk jug, and fill the balance of the jug with water. Stir, and add ½ cup of the mixture to every gallon of water you use to water your container plants.

## Yard & Garden

● Your holiday houseplants will stay chipper all season long if you feed them with this solution: 1 gallon of water mixed with ¼ cup of beer and ½ tablespoon each of unflavored gelatin, Fish Emulsion, Vitamin $B_1$ Plant Starter, ammonia, and instant tea granules.

● To get your seeds off to a disease-free start, lightly sprinkle flavored gelatin powder on them with a salt shaker. Any flavor will work, but lemon is best because it repels some bugs.

● As your young plants grow, feed them every couple of weeks with flavored gelatin mix. Gently work a tablespoon or so of the powder into the soil, being careful not to disturb the roots. The gelatin itself helps the soil hold water, and the sugar feeds the micro-organisms in the soil.

# GIZMOS & GADGETS

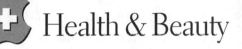 Health & Beauty

Use ice cube trays to freeze your favorite skin lotion (homemade or store-bought). That way, you'll always have cool, soothing relief on hand for sunburn, chapped skin, or insect bites.

Protect a bandaged finger and keep the area dry by pulling an uninflated balloon over it before you tackle a wet job like washing the car, the dishes, or the dog.

Do you break a nail every time you open an aspirin bottle? Save your nails (and your good humor) by keeping a bottle opener right next to the aspirin—or any other bottle that has a hard-to-pop top.

Make toothpaste last longer by squeezing the end of the tube with a large binder clip from the supermarket stationery section. (This same trick works just as well for ointments, creams, hair gels, and even kitchen condiments that come in tubes.)

Tuck a muffin tin into your bathroom vanity drawer to hold the small stuff that tends to accumulate there like safety pins, trial-size bottles and tubes, and tiny jars of cosmetics.

## TRASH TO TREASURE

**WHAT DO you do with extra kitchen gadgets—say, your third set of measuring cups, or that extra egg timer that's buried in the junk drawer? Use them as the start of a child's private treasure chest. Find a nifty, old wooden box, or maybe a giant-sized tin that once held popcorn, and toss in all those supermarket gizmos that go bang or clang, hold sand or water, or just look neat. This list will give you some ideas:**

- ○ **Colander**
- ○ **Ice cream scoop**
- ○ **Measuring spoons**
- ○ **Salad spinner**
- ○ **Wooden spoons**

◉ Here's another bathroom storage idea that comes from the kitchen—or, rather, the kitchen-gadget section at the supermarket: Get a few of those wire hanging baskets that are meant to store produce, and hang them from the bathroom ceiling. They're perfect for stashing soap, extra toilet paper, and all sorts of health and beauty gear.

# Home Cleaning & Upkeep

◆ Crack! Splat! There goes an egg off the counter and onto the floor. How are you going to get rid of *that* mess? With a turkey baster, that's how! It'll swoop that eggy goo right up.

◆ Avoid spills when filling a steam iron by using a turkey baster to get the liquid into the iron.

◆ Is your necklace collection a tangled pile in the bottom of your jewelry box? Here's a quick fix that's as close as your supermarket's gadget section: Get a wooden coat hanger and a package of cup hooks (or larger mug hooks if your chains are on the chunky side). Screw the hooks into the coat hanger, hang up your necklaces, and presto—end of clutter!

◆ Organize rings, pins, and earrings by keeping them in plastic ice cube trays.

◆ Here's a timesaving cleaning tip: Keep a rubber band around each container of furniture polish or spray cleaner. What for? To hold a soft cloth or sponge. That way, you'll always have one when you need it!

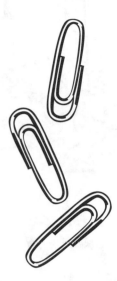

◆ Ironing a pleated skirt will be a breeze if you hold the pleats in place with bobby pins or paper clips.

◆ Got some new, leather-soled shoes? Before you wear them for the first time, roughen up the soles with an emery board to prevent slips and falls.

◆ Raise the nap on suede shoes or jackets by rubbing the spots gently with the smoother side of an emery board. (Don't use a metal nail file; it could damage the suede.)

◆ Use a soft paintbrush to dust baskets, wicker furniture, or anything with tiny gaps and crevices that are hard to reach with a cloth.

◆ Use photo albums from the supermarket stationery section to organize recipes, business cards, and other small, but important papers. Albums with clear plastic pockets work best because you can slide the contents in and out for easy rearrangement.

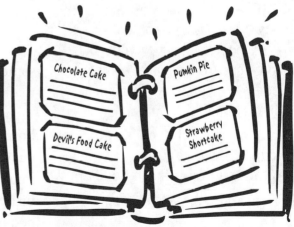

◆ When you lose the pull tab on a zipper, replace it with a small paper clip or safety pin. Disguise the little gadget by giving it a dab of paint, or by wrapping it in thread that matches the color of the garment.

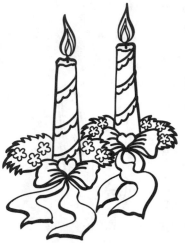

◆ Want to add pizzazz to plain candles? Use a vegetable peeler to carve designs in the wax.

◆ Tired of licking envelopes at bill-paying time? Lick the problem by sealing the flaps with a dampened pastry brush.

## Kids & Pets

■ Here's a great wading-pool or tub toy for a child or grandchild: a turkey baster. Once they get the hang of it, tiny tykes will spend hours on end making the water go in and out.

■ Is there an infant in the house? Tuck a few ice cube trays into a dresser drawer to corral baby socks and booties.

■ Want to give a small child some rainy-day fun? Buy the biggest foil roasting pan or Styrofoam® cooler your supermarket has, and fill it almost to the brim with dried beans. Toss in measuring cups, a funnel, and a few well-rinsed lids from detergent bottles. Now you've got a first-class entertainment center for anybody between the ages of about 3 and 6. (That's old enough not to swallow the beans, but young enough to enjoy tossing them around.)

### REMARKABLE RECIPES

### PUP-SICLES

For hot-weather treats—or to distract a teething puppy from your favorite sneakers—gather some ice cube trays, and make a few batches of these goodies.

**½ cup of finely chopped vegetables**
**½ cup of plain yogurt**
**1 qt. of beef or chicken bouillon**

Mix all of the ingredients together, and pour the mixture into ice cube trays. Then tuck them into the freezer until treat time rolls around.

■ If your kids or grandkids are going through that stage where they love teeny-tiny toys, give them a bunch of ice cube trays to keep their treasures in.

■ Here's the problem: You need to transport a small animal, you don't have a pet carrier, and there's no time to get one from a pet shop. Here's the simple solution: Put the critter inside a plastic laundry basket, invert another one over it (make sure both baskets are the same size), and tie the edges together. Bingo—you're ready to go!

# Workshop & Garage

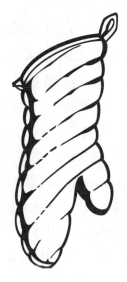

▼ Stash a pair of oven mitts in your car for those times when you need to touch hot or messy car parts.

▼ Save time and hassle by keeping a plastic laundry basket in the trunk of your car. Then, when you're out shopping, put your packages in the basket. That way, they won't get tossed about, and when you get home, you can tote the whole load into the house in one trip.

▼ When a key breaks off in your car's trunk or door lock, don't call a locksmith—at least, not right away. First, try to work the broken piece free using a curved tapestry needle. (You'll find them in the supermarket's sewing section.)

▼ To keep a skin from forming on the paint in a partially used can, blow up a balloon, and push it into the can before you put the lid on.

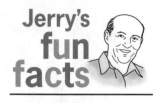

In 1916, Clarence Saunders opened the world's first self-service grocery store in Memphis, Tennessee. He called it Piggly Wiggly. Folks thought the concept was crazy. (At that time, shoppers gave their list to a clerk, who gathered the goods and met the customer at the front counter.) Well, I'd say the idea is here to stay. The name has hung around, too, with some 600 Piggly Wiggly stores in 16 states.

▼ Do you need to paint a ceiling, or some overhead woodwork? Here's a great trick for catching those annoying drips: Get a hollow rubber ball from the supermarket toy section. Slice the ball in half, cut a slit in one of the halves, and slide it over your paint-brush handle, hollow side up. You'll finish the job with paint-free hair and arms!

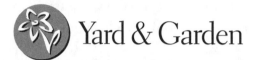

# Yard & Garden

● Use plastic ice cube trays as seed-starter flats. Just poke a few drainage holes in the bottom of each compartment, fill them with seed-starting mix, and plant your seeds. Set the trays in a shallow pan, and you're off to the races!

● Give the birds a winter water supply using a 12-inch-diameter plastic storage bowl with a snap-on lid. Here's how: Spray both the bowl and lid with flat black enamel. When the paint dries, cut or drill a 1-inch-diameter hole in the lid, fill the bowl with water, and set it in a sunny spot. The black color will absorb and hold the sun's heat, so a layer of water will remain, even in freezing weather. Check often, and keep the water high enough so the birds can reach it through the hole in the lid.

● To drain water from plant saucers, or to water hanging plants the easy way, use a turkey baster.

● Is your garage or shed cluttered with small tools, twine, plant labels, and other small garden gear? Tidy up the place by stashing that stuff in a hanging shoe bag from the supermarket's housewares section.

# GREEN TEA

 ## Health & Beauty

❡ Make a skin toner by mixing 1 teaspoon of green tea leaves with ½ cup of witch hazel. Dab it onto your face with a cotton pad—no need to rinse.

❡ You forgot to wear your hat to the ballgame and wound up with a sunburned scalp? This will ease the pain: Brew a pot of green tea. While it's cooling, wash your hair with a gentle shampoo, and rinse with the cool tea.

❡ Do your choppers a favor: Drink a cup of green tea after every meal. It contains tooth-friendly tannin, which kills decay-causing bacteria and stops them from producing glucans, the sticky substance that helps bacteria cling to your teeth.

❡ Want to cut your risk of cancer? (Of course you do! Who doesn't?) Then drink plenty of green tea. Medical studies show that it contains the strongest known form of antioxidants, and that consuming four to six cups a day seems to reduce the incidence of all sorts of cancer, as well as protect against heart disease and rheumatoid arthritis.

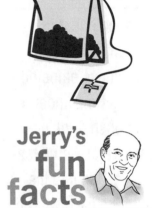

**Jerry's fun facts**

Here's good news for those of you who don't care much for the taste of green tea, or who don't want to consume caffeine: You can get all of the health benefits, without caffeine, by taking green tea pills. They're available in the vitamin or health-food section of most big supermarkets.

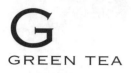

## Jerry's fun facts

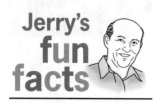

Legend has it that around 2700 B.C., a Chinese emperor was sitting under a tea bush drinking hot water. Some tea leaves fell into his cup, he liked what he tasted, and bingo— a beverage made from unfermented, a.k.a. green, tea leaves was born.

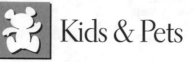

## Kids & Pets

■ If your dog breaks out in hot spots—red, wet skin eruptions—take him to the vet as soon as you can. In the meantime, relieve his discomfort with a poultice of cool, moist green tea bags. Apply them directly to the spots, and hold them on for as long as Spot's patience holds out.

■ Does Fido have chronic skin problems? The most likely cause is a food allergy, so to give him long-term relief, see a holistic vet. In the meantime, though, ease his discomfort by giving him a green tea bath. Just brew up enough to fill a basin, let it cool, and saturate his coat, making sure that the liquid reaches the skin. Don't rinse; just let the tea do its therapeutic work. (The amount of tea you'll need will depend on the dog's size, but figure on 1 teabag per cup of water.)

■ Help protect your pets from cancer, which is on the rise in dogs and cats, by adding green tea to their diet. You can either give it to them in pill form, or mix the tea leaves into their food. (Consult a holistic vet for precise dosages, but when in doubt, don't worry: It's impossible to deliver an overdose!)

■ Comfort a child who's just had a shot by applying a wet green tea bag to the scene of the "crime."

# GROCERY BAGS

## 🏠 Home Cleaning & Upkeep

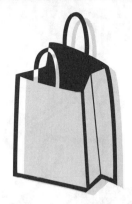

◆ Empty your bagless, hand-held vacuum cleaner inside a brown paper grocery bag. That way, the dust won't fly all over the room. To dispose of the dirt, just throw the bag and contents on the compost pile.

◆ Make a fire starter by stuffing a small brown paper bag with newspaper and a few candle nubbins.

◆ Turn a brown paper grocery bag into a useful work of art. Paint designs on it, or cover it with pictures cut from magazines or wrapping paper. Give it a couple coats of clear acrylic enamel, inside and out, and presto: a decorative wastebasket, magazine holder, dried-flower vase—or a container for who-knows-what.

◆ Need an emergency pressing cloth? Cut open a brown paper grocery bag along the seams, dampen it, and use it just as you would a piece of ordinary fabric.

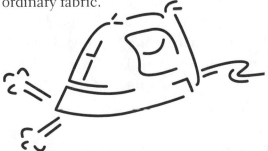

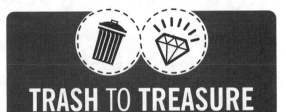

## TRASH TO TREASURE

**EVEN AFTER you've used a plastic grocery bag a few times, there could be a lot of life left in it. In fact, if you tuck that bag into a recycling bin at the supermarket, it will be processed into wood-polymer lumber that's used for making hardworking structures like boardwalks, nature trails, decks, and outdoor furniture. That means the bag you carry home today could very well be a seat you'll be sitting on a few months from now!**

## Kids & Pets

■ Put plastic grocery bags to work as pooper scoopers. Tuck a few into your pocket when you take your pooch for a walk. When he does his duty, pick the stuff up with the bag, flip it inside out, and tie it closed. (They also work great for dispensing with scooped-up, clumping cat litter.)

■ If you like to make playthings for your kids or grandkids, this idea's for you: Use plastic grocery bags as waterproof stuffing for vinyl or terrycloth kiddie-pool and bathtub toys. (Crumpled-up bags make dandy outdoor-cushion innards, too.)

■ Got a kids' party coming up? Create streamers by cutting colorful plastic bags into strips. Start at the open end, and stop when you get within about 2 inches of the bottom. Hang the bags from cord that you've strung on the wall or across the ceiling.

■ Make Halloween masks from brown paper bags. Cut eye, nose, and mouth holes, then let the kids go to town decorating them with paints, crayons, felt-tip markers, sequins, glitter, or whatever suits their fancy.

## TRASH TO TREASURE

HERE'S A way to make sure you always have a neat-looking supply of plastic bags at your finger tips: Each time you empty a box of facial tissue, hang on to it. When you get home from the grocery store, stuff your plastic grocery bags into the box. That stash will come in mighty handy in the kitchen, garage, tool shed, trunk of your car—or just about anyplace else!

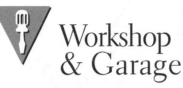

## Workshop & Garage

▼ If you have to leave your car outdoors overnight in the winter, keep the windshield free of snow and ice this way: Cut a brown paper bag apart, spread it across the windshield, and secure it in place with the wiper blades. Come morning, strip off the bag, and toss it on the compost pile or into the recycling bin.

▼ When the summer sun is baking and you can't find your windshield protector, use a brown paper bag instead. Just cut it apart, lay it against the inside of the windshield, and lower the visors to hold it to the glass.

## Yard & Garden

● Add brown paper bags to your compost pile—they're a perfect source of necessary carbon. Run the bags through a paper shredder for almost-instant breakdown, or simply crumple them up and toss them onto the heap.

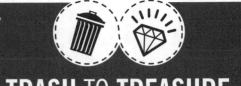

## TRASH TO TREASURE

HERE'S A handful of ideas for reusing both paper and plastic grocery bags around the house:

○ Pack your lunch (paper or plastic)

○ Cover textbooks (paper)

○ Wrap Christmas, birthday, or party gifts (paper)

○ Ripen fruit more quickly (paper)

○ Line trash cans (plastic)

○ Dispose of used cat litter (plastic)

○ "Waterproof" flashlights and radios on camping and boating trips (plastic; keep 'em under wraps, even while in use)

○ Take the place of those expensive flannel bags some folks buy to pack their shoes in when they travel (plastic)

# G

## GROCERY BAGS

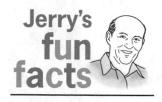
● Use brown paper bags to help ease your garden cleanup chores. Just set one beside you whenever you're deadheading flowers or pruning healthy plants. When the bag is full, throw it and its contents onto the compost pile. (Never compost diseased plant material; either burn it or send it off with the trash collector.)

● Get rid of weeds with brown paper bags. Trample tall weeds or, if you like, mow them down. Then spread your bags on top, overlapping as you go, until the layer is three or four bags deep. If you're making a path or walkway, add gravel or another foot-friendly substance. To make an instant planting bed, pile on 6 to 8 inches of topsoil and compost.

● Trap borers and other tree-damaging pests by wrapping brown paper bags around the tree's trunk—overlapping and taping them together as you go—and coating the paper with petroleum jelly or a commercial adhesive. (Remember to check your traps every week or so, and replace them with new ones.)

● Turn plastic grocery bags into scarecrows. Fill them with air, tie them shut, and fasten them to the top of stakes about 5 to 6 feet tall. Push the stakes into the ground in a random pattern, 10 to 15 feet apart, throughout your garden. When the bags bob in the breeze, they look an awful lot like people bending over, and birds don't like that one little bit!

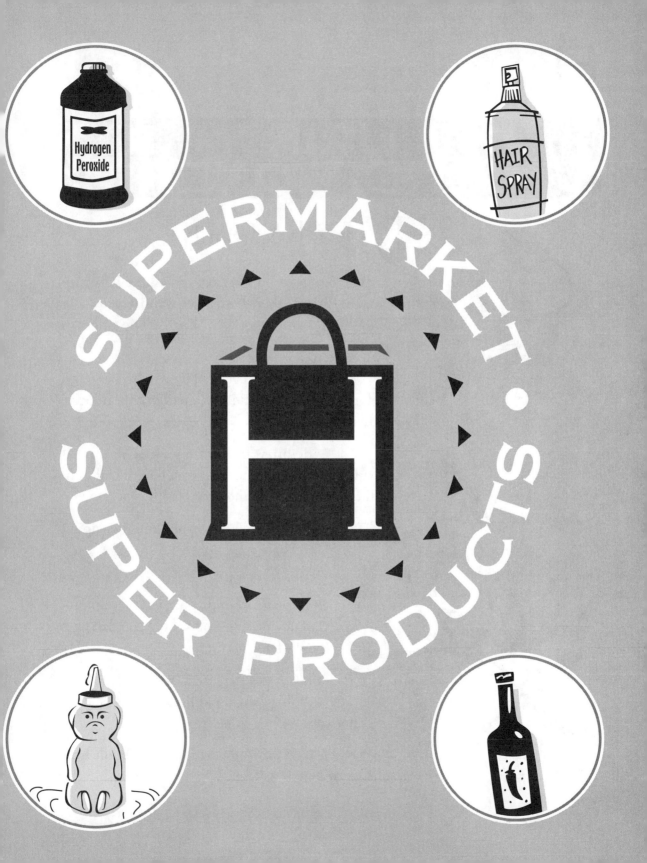

# H

# HAIR CONDITIONER

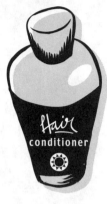

## ⚕ Health & Beauty

To remove a tight ring, rub a little hair conditioner on the finger, then hold your hand toward the ceiling to let fluid drain out of your fingers. The ring will slide right off.

To soften your feet, coat them with hair conditioner before you go to bed. Pull on a pair of cotton socks, and wear them overnight.

Before you take a dip in a chlorinated pool, rub a little conditioner into your hair. It will minimize the drying effect of the pool chemicals.

Soften chapped hands by wiping on a little hair conditioner.

Dab a little hair conditioner on the skin around your eyes to help prevent dry lines. Just make sure you don't get the stuff *in* your eyes!

Soothe freshly shaved legs by rubbing hair conditioner into the skin after your shower or bath.

A drop or two of hair conditioner on a tissue or cotton ball gently removes makeup.

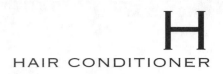

 Before you remove an adhesive bandage, lift up each side just a little, and rub a drop of hair conditioner onto the spot where it meets the skin. Wait a few minutes, then peel off the bandage—painlessly.

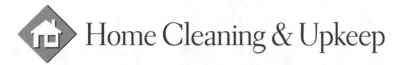

# Home Cleaning & Upkeep

◆ Clean and polish silver with hair conditioner. Just pour a little onto a clean, soft cotton cloth, and rub a thin coat onto the dry silver. Gently wipe off the excess. A very thin, virtually invisible coating will stay behind, and actually protect the silver from tarnishing!

◆ To keep drawers, windows, and sliding doors from sticking, lubricate their tracks with hair conditioner.

◆ Got a faucet that's screeching? Remove the handle and stem, coat both sets of the metal threads with hair conditioner, and put the pieces back in place.

◆ Coat the edges of refrigerator racks with a thin layer of hair conditioner. They'll slide easily every time.

◆ Put the hush on squeaky door hinges by adding a drop or two of hair conditioner to the moving parts.

◆ Keep shower curtains gliding easily by applying a thin coat of hair conditioner to the curtain rod.

◆ Hide scratches on wood furniture or paneling. Pour a few drops of hair conditioner on a clean, soft cotton cloth, rub the wood, and buff with a second cloth.

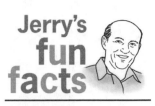

**Jerry's fun facts**

I don't know whether blondes really have more fun than other folks, but they do have more hair, conditioned or not. On average, the head of a blonde-haired person (natural blonde, that is) has 140,000 individual hairs. Folks with brown or black hair average 110,000 strands, and redheads have roughly 90,000 hairs.

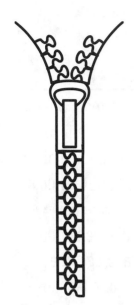

♦ Make a stainless steel sink sparkle with a dab of hair conditioner on a soft cloth.

♦ Zippers slide easily when you rub a little hair conditioner on the teeth.

♦ Clean and condition leather with hair conditioner. Just rub it on and buff with a soft cotton cloth.

♦ Shoes squeaking? Dribble a drop or two of hair conditioner onto the trouble spots.

 ## Kids & Pets

■ To break in a new fielder's mitt, rub it with hair conditioner, tuck a baseball where the future pocket will be, and fold the glove around it. Secure it with a belt, and tuck it under your little slugger's mattress overnight.

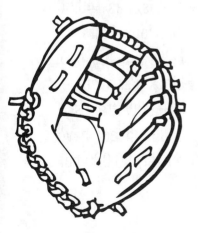

■ Lubricate bike chains, roller skates, and skateboard wheels with a few drops of hair conditioner.

■ In winter, before you take your dog for a walk on de-iced sidewalks, rub his paws with hair conditioner. It will help keep salt and other chemicals from irritating his foot pads. When you get back inside, wash Fido's paws (including the hair between his toes) with dog shampoo and rinse thoroughly—before he has a chance to lick off any of the toxic chemicals.

■ To shine a horse's hooves, rub in a little hair conditioner, and buff with a clean cloth.

■ The same conditioner you use on your hair will detangle a horse's mane and tail. Just rub a little through the strands, and comb as usual.

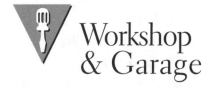

# Workshop & Garage

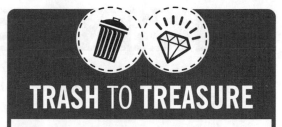

## TRASH TO TREASURE

**BEFORE YOU** toss that hair conditioner bottle into the recycling bin, fill it about halfway with warm water, give it a good shake, and put it right back into the bathroom. Even though the contents are watery, the conditioning power is still there. You'll get a few more hair treatments out of it, for sure.

▼ At painting time, coat any hinges, doorknobs, lock latches, and window pulls with hair conditioner. That way, the paint won't stick to the surfaces, and all you'll have to do to clean up is wipe the hardware with a soft cloth.

▼ Does paint always seem to wind up in your hair? Before you start a painting job, pour a quarter-sized dab of hair conditioner onto your head, and slick it through your hair. The paint will wash out more easily.

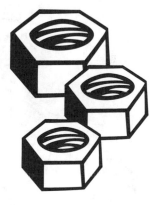

▼ Before you undertake a messy job like fixing the car or painting, lightly coat your hands with hair conditioner. When your work is through, those dirty mitts will come clean without hard scrubbing or harsh solvents.

▼ Nuts, bolts, and pipe connections will fit together easily—and not rust together later—when you lubricate them with conditioner *before* you screw them in place.

▼ Keep your tools from rusting by rubbing on a light coat of hair conditioner.

# H

# HAIR SPRAY

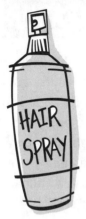

### 🏠 Home Cleaning & Upkeep

◆ Ink stains on upholstery fabric? Grab two thick, white towels. Spritz one with hair spray, and leave the other one dry. Alternately dab the stains with the sprayed towel and the dry one until the marks are gone.

◆ To get rid of ink stains on clothing, spray the spots with hair spray, and launder as usual.

◆ Make pantyhose (especially the sandalfoot kind) last longer by spraying the heels and toes of each new pair with hair spray. If you've already got a run in your hose, keep it from spreading by zapping it with hair spray.

◆ Spray new canvas sneakers with hair spray to keep them looking like new longer.

◆ You sewing buffs will find it easier to thread your needle if you stiffen the end of the thread with hair spray first.

◆ A light coat of hair spray will keep newly polished brass from tarnishing.

◆ Hair spray makes a perfect light adhesive for all sorts of craft projects.

◆ Make an inexpensive gift wrap by spraying the Sunday comics with hair spray. It seals in the ink and gives the paper a nice gloss. (Kids love it, too!)

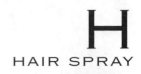

◆ Before you hang a wreath outside, spray the ribbons and bows with super-hold hair spray, and let it dry. They'll stay clean and perky. (Just don't hang them where they'll get rained on, or the hair spray will wash off.)

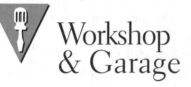

## Workshop & Garage

▼ Having trouble putting new rubber grips on your bike's handle-bars? Spray the inside of the new grip with hair spray. It works as a lubricant when it's wet, but it dries like glue to keep the grips in place.

▼ In a workshop, project diagrams and how-to instructions can get grimy fast. Keep them clean and read-able by coating them with hair spray.

## Yard & Garden

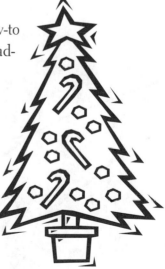

● Your Christmas tree will keep its nee-dles longer if you give them a light coat of hair spray within the first day or two of bringing the tree inside.

● Cut flowers will last longer if you spray them with hair spray *after* they've been in the vase for a day or so.

---

**TRASH TO TREASURE**

IF YOU use a hair spray that comes in a pump bottle rather than an aerosol can, hang on to those bottles! Washed and rinsed, they're perfect for holding garden tonics, homemade spray cleaners, or even food-coloring "spray paint" for the kids. (See page 121 for an easy paint recipe.)

# H

# HAND & BODY LOTION

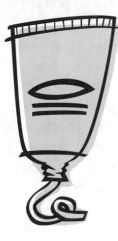

## 🍎➕ Health & Beauty

🍎 Add some hand & body lotion to your shampoo to help moisturize your hair each time you wash it.

🍎 Use lotion to style your hair. Just rub a generous amount between your hands, smooth it onto your hair, and arrange it in the "do" that you want.

🍎 Make a moisturizing sunscreen by mixing hand & body lotion with sunblock.

🍎 When you open a new bottle of nail polish, run a little lotion along the outside rim of the bottle. The next time you open it, the top won't stick.

🍎 Got a ring stuck on your finger? Coat the digit with lotion, and the ring should slide right off.

🍎 Fresh out of shaving cream? Don't run to the store—use hand & body lotion instead.

🍎 Hey, guys! This tip's just for you—that is, if you sport a beard that picks up static when the air turns cold and dry. You can end those flyaway frizzies by mixing a little hand & body lotion with a drop of water in your palm, and rubbing the mixture into your beard.

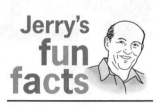

## Home Cleaning & Upkeep

◆ To eliminate static cling on slips or panty-hose, rub hand & body lotion into your hands until it disappears, then run your palms over the troublesome clothing.

◆ Shine your shoes with a dab of hand & body lotion on a soft cotton cloth. Buff thoroughly.

◆ Use hand & body lotion on your hands before you put on rubber gloves, and they'll slide on more easily.

◆ Before your kids or grandkids (or even grown-ups!) spend time outside on a cold, windy day, apply a thick layer of hand & body lotion on cheeks to prevent chapping.

## Kids & Pets

■ If you've ever tried putting those tight water shoes on the feet of a wiggly child, you know how difficult it can be. Here's help: Smear some hand & body lotion (or sunscreen) on those tiny tootsies, and the water shoes will slide right on!

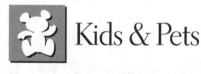

# H

# HONEY

## Health & Beauty

To banish blackheads, heat a little honey, and apply it directly to the affected areas. Let it sit for a minute or two, wash it off with warm water, then rinse with cool water. Pat dry.

For a smooth, silky bath, add ¼ cup of honey to the water as you're filling the tub.

Here's a sweet recipe for a softening facial: Thoroughly combine 2 tablespoons of honey, 2 tablespoons of mashed avocado, and 1 egg yolk. Apply the mixture to your face. Leave it on for 30 minutes or so, rinse with warm water, and pat dry.

Want an even simpler skin treatment? Just mash a banana, and add 1 tablespoon of honey. Cover your face with the mixture, let it sit for 15 minutes, then rinse with warm water.

Yes, you have no bananas? Substitute a peeled and cored apple in the mixture above, and purée it with 1 tablespoon of honey. Smooth the mix on your face, and leave it on for 15 minutes. Then rinse with warm water.

### REMARKABLE RECIPES

### HONEY & CUCUMBER CLEANSER

When you want to soothe and revitalize your skin at the same time, whip up this simple lotion.

**¼ of a small cucumber, peeled and seeded**
**2 tbsp. of honey**
**1 tbsp. of whole milk**

Purée the cucumber, strain it, and pour its juice into a bowl. Mix in the honey, add the milk, and stir. Using cotton pads, apply the mixture to your face and neck. Wait 20 minutes, then rinse.

🍎 If you just want to get down to basics, try this neat treat: Add 2 tablespoons of honey to 1 cup of warm water, and mix well. Smooth the honey-water onto your face, let it sit for about 30 minutes, and rinse it off.

🍎 For a honey of a hair conditioner, mix 1 tablespoon of honey and 2 tablespoons of olive oil. Warm the mixture, dip your fingers into it, and rub it into the strands of your hair. Soak a towel in hot water, wring it out completely, and wrap it around your head. Leave it in place for 20 minutes, and shampoo as usual, lathering well to remove the oil.

🍎 To make your pearly whites whiter, brush them with a mixture of 1 tablespoon of honey and 1 tablespoon of charcoal. (Make sure you get charcoal that's made for horticultural and aquarium use—*not* the kind made for barbecue grills!)

🍎 A dab of honey takes the itch out of bee stings.

🍎 Tickle in your throat? Put a tablespoon or two of honey into a cup of hot water, add a teaspoon of lemon juice, stir well, and drink to your health. Repeat every few hours, and your sore throat should be gone in a day or two. (If it's not, call your doctor.)

🍎 If you prefer to take your medicine straight, sip 1 tablespoon of honey at bedtime, and let it trickle down your throat. For best results, warm the honey first so that it flows smoothly.

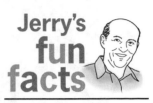

**Jerry's fun facts**

Here are a few things I'll bet you didn't know about our honey-making, buzzin' buddies:

• The first honeybees to hit our shores arrived with European colonists around 1638.

• On average, it takes the lifetime labor of 12 bees to produce just 1 teaspoon of honey.

• A hive of bees must fly more than 55,000 miles and tap about 2 million flowers to produce 1 pound of honey.

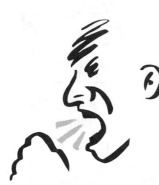

To relieve a cough due to a cold, dissolve 1 teaspoon of honey and 1 tablespoon of lemon juice in a small glass of warm water, and sip it. For a stronger solution, combine equal parts of honey and lemon, and take 1 teaspoon at bedtime. Either mixture will help loosen phlegm.

When you need to cure a hangover, don't take the hair of the dog—take the juice of the bee. Honey, a concentrated source of fructose, will help your system flush out whatever alcohol remains in your body. Just spread the honey on toast or crackers, and eat up.

## REMARKABLE RECIPES

### SOOTHING SUNBURN BATH

Kids love this foaming bath, even when they don't have sunburned skin. (Grown-ups go for it, too!)

**1 cup of vegetable oil**
**½ cup of honey**
**½ cup of liquid hand soap**
**1 tbsp. of pure vanilla extract (not artificial)**

Mix all of the ingredients together, and pour the mixture into a bottle with a tight stopper. At bath time, shake the bottle, then pour ¼ cup or so under running water.

## Kids & Pets

A teaspoon of honey at bedtime helps children sleep through the night—and helps solve bed-wetting problems. The sweet stuff acts as a sedative, and attracts and holds fluid in the child's body. One word of caution: *Never* give honey to a baby under 2 years of age.

When a child gets a minor bump or scrape, dab a little honey on it. Because honey is hygroscopic (that is, it absorbs water), it deprives infection-causing microorganisms of the moisture they need to survive. Best of all from the victim's standpoint, though, honey won't sting the way some antiseptics do.

# HOT PEPPERS & HOT SAUCE

## 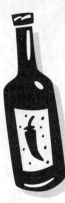 Health & Beauty

Want to give yourself a healthy "high"? Just eat something that's spiced up with chile peppers. To counteract the chiles' heat, your brain releases chemicals called endorphins, which give you a sense of pleasure and well-being.

Has too much time at the computer left you with a sore shoulder? Make your own pain-relief ointment by adding 3 to 4 drops of hot pepper sauce to 2 teaspoons of olive oil. Massage the ointment into your shoulder three or four times a day.

Relieve a toothache by rubbing a drop or two of hot pepper sauce onto the gum at the base of your achy tooth.

Coming down with a cold? Three or four times a day, mix 10 to 20 drops of hot pepper sauce or a big pinch of cayenne pepper in a glass of tomato juice, and drink to your health.

Sore throat? Substitute water for the tomato juice (see above), and gargle several times a day.

Besides clearing your sinuses and soothing your throat, cayenne helps keep your heart muscle in good shape. So eat it every chance you get!

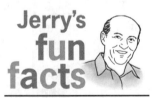

**Jerry's fun facts**

During the 1980s, teenagers in New York City took to sucking subway tokens out of the turnstiles. How did the cops stop the rascals? They sprinkled hot pepper on the token slots!

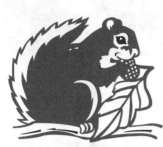

## Yard & Garden

● To keep squirrels from clearing out your bird feeder, mix a tablespoon or so of ground cayenne in with the birdseed.

● If it's your tulips the squirrels are after, try this tactic: Mix 3 tablespoons of cayenne pepper with 2 cups of hot water in a bottle, and shake well. Let it sit overnight, strain off the liquid, and mix it in a hand-held spray bottle with 1 tablespoon each of hot sauce, ammonia, and baby shampoo. Start spraying the stems when the flowers appear, and continue as long as new buds are forming.

● Cabbage pests on the rampage? Mix 2 tablespoons of cayenne pepper with 1 cup of flour, and dust the results on all your cabbage-family plants. Cabbageworms and loopers will eat the mixture and die; other bad guys will simply go elsewhere when they smell (or taste) the pepper.

● Here's a potent spray for all kinds of leaf-eating bugs: Combine four to six garlic cloves, one small onion, and two hot peppers (or 1 teaspoon of ground cayenne) in a blender with 1 quart of water, and liquefy. Let it sit overnight, strain out the solids, and add 3 drops of baby shampoo. Pour the solution into a hand-held spray bottle, and you're good to go.

### REMARKABLE RECIPES

### DOG-BE-GONE TONIC

Keep roaming dogs out of your yard with this spicy potion.

**2 cloves of garlic**
**2 small onions**
**1 jalapeño pepper**
**1 tbsp. of cayenne pepper**
**1 tbsp. of Tabasco® sauce**
**1 tbsp. of chili powder**
**1 tbsp. of dishwashing liquid**
**1 qt. of warm water**

Chop the garlic, onions, and jalapeño, and combine them with the rest of the ingredients. Let the mixture sit for 24 hours, then strain out the solids, and sprinkle the solution on any areas where dogs are a problem.

# HYDROGEN PEROXIDE

## Health & Beauty

🍎 Make your own whitening toothpaste by combining hydrogen peroxide with just enough baking soda to make a paste.

🍎 To clear up a persistent case of gingivitis, use this gum paste. Shake about 1 teaspoon of baking soda into a small dish, and drizzle in just enough hydrogen peroxide to make a paste. Gently work it under the gum line with your toothbrush. Leave the paste on for a few minutes, then rinse well with cool water.

🍎 Freshen and clean your toothbrush by letting it soak overnight in a cup filled with enough hydrogen peroxide to cover the bristles. Rinse the brush before using it.

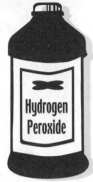

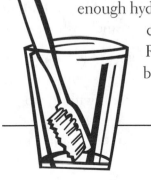

**REMARKABLE RECIPES**

### HALITOSIS HELPER

Good old peroxide is great for curing bad breath. And the recipe couldn't be easier!

**Hydrogen peroxide**
**Water**
**Flavored oil (optional)**

Mix equal parts hydrogen peroxide and water in a cup, and swish in your mouth. Do not swallow! Spit it out, and rinse your mouth again with cool water. If the taste of hydrogen peroxide doesn't suit you, add a drop or two of flavored oil, such as peppermint, to the mouthwash.

## Home Cleaning & Upkeep

◆ Clean the grout on ceramic-tile walls and floors with an old toothbrush dipped into a paste made of equal parts hydrogen peroxide and baking soda.

◆ If your store-bought, scratchless scrubbing powder doesn't do the trick on tough stains, give it a boost with this formula. Make a paste out of the cleanser and some fresh hydrogen peroxide (check the date on the bottle). Add a pinch of cream of tartar. Leave this poultice on the stain for 30 minutes, then scrub it off with a brush or a scouring sponge. Caution: *Never* combine hydrogen peroxide with any substance that contains any chlorine!

◆ Linens that have been stored for a long time can become yellowed with age. But don't use bleach to clean them; it can damage the fabric. Instead, sponge the spots with hydrogen peroxide or, if the whole piece is yellowed, submerge it in the peroxide. Either way, let it sit for an hour or so, rinse with cold water, and wash as usual.

◆ Got grass or dirt stains on white cotton clothes? Before you wash the garments, pre-treat the spots with hydrogen peroxide. (It's gentler than bleach on cotton fibers.) Let it sit on the stain for a few minutes before washing.

◆ Hydrogen peroxide is great for removing blood stains from light-colored fabrics. Just pre-treat the stain before laundering.

◆ Wash toxic chemicals from fruits and vegetables with hydrogen peroxide, and rinse with clear water.

 ## Yard & Garden

● Keep your herb garden healthy by feeding the plants every six weeks with this mixture: 1 cup of tea and ½ tablespoon each of hydrogen peroxide, bourbon, and ammonia in 1 gallon of warm water.

● In the fall, when you dig up your tender bulbs, wash them in a solution of 2 tablespoons of baby shampoo and 1 teaspoon of hydrogen peroxide mixed in a quart of warm water. Make sure you dry the bulbs thoroughly before you store them for the winter.

● Protect your roses and other mildew-prone plants by spraying them every week in the spring with a mix of 1 tablespoon of hydrogen peroxide, 1 tablespoon of baby shampoo, 1 teaspoon of instant tea granules, and 2 cups of water in a hand-held spray bottle.

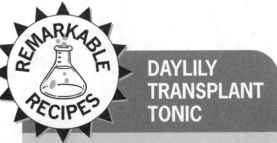

**REMARKABLE RECIPES**

## DAYLILY TRANSPLANT TONIC

When you divide daylilies or other perennial favorites, get the transplanted divisions off to a good start with this elixir.

**½ can of beer
2 tbsp. of dishwashing liquid
2 tbsp. of ammonia
2 tbsp. of Fish Emulsion
1 tbsp. of hydrogen peroxide
¼ tsp. of instant tea granules
2 gal. of water**

Mix all of these ingredients in a large bucket. Just before setting the plants into their new homes, pour 2 cups of the mixture into each hole.

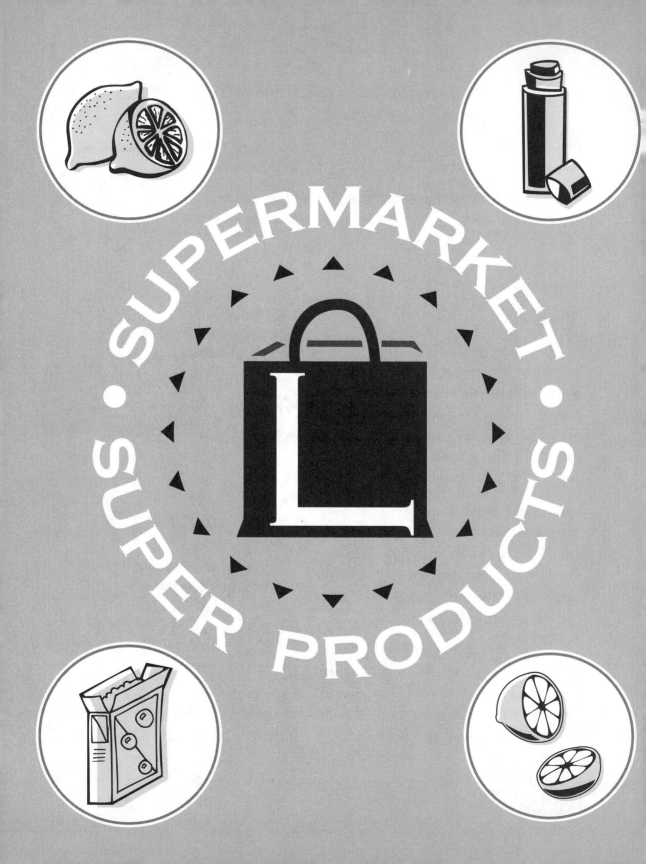

# LAUNDRY DETERGENT

## 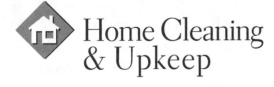 Health & Beauty

When a messy chore leaves you with greasy, oily hands, wash them with laundry detergent. They'll be clean as a whistle in no time!

To clean your hairbrushes, fill the bathroom sink with warm water and add 1 tablespoon of laundry detergent and ½ cup of borax. Swish the brushes around in the sudsy water several times, rinse in clear water, and let them dry.

## Home Cleaning & Upkeep

Could your wicker furniture use a good cleaning? Put about 1 tablespoon of mild laundry detergent in 4 cups of warm water, and mix until frothy. Apply the suds to the furniture with a soft cloth, working one area at a time. Wipe with a clean, damp cloth.

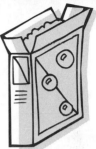

**REMARKABLE RECIPES**

### ALL-PURPOSE CLEANUP MIX

Here's a handy recipe that you can use on stucco, concrete, or any other outdoor surface.

⅓ cup of powdered laundry detergent
⅔ cup of powdered household detergent (like Spic and Span®)
1 gal. of water

Mix all of the ingredients together, put on a pair of rubber gloves, grab a sponge, and you're ready to go. Use a stiff-bristle brush to scrub stubborn stains. If you're cleaning something that's mildewy, use less water and add about a pint of bleach to the mix.

◆ Clean decks, porches, and wood fences with a solution made of ½ cup of powdered laundry detergent and 1 quart of bleach in 2 gallons of water. Scrub the surface using a stiff broom or brush, and rinse thoroughly with the garden hose.

◆ Vinyl or aluminum siding will stay new-looking for years if you follow this annual routine: First, give the siding a good, strong spray from a garden hose. Then, go at any spots with a scrub brush and a solution of ¼ cup of powdered laundry detergent and 2 gallons of water. Rinse well when you're done.

## TRASH TO TREASURE

**NEED AN extra watering can?** Don't go out and buy a new one—recycle an old laundry detergent bottle instead. Start with a giant-sized bottle that has a handle. Wash it out thoroughly, drill 10 or 12 holes in the cap (or as many as you have room for), and let the $H_2O$ flow! If you use a brightly colored bottle, your new can will have an added advantage: You won't lose track of it in the garden.

## Yard & Garden

● When you feed your lawn, give the fertilizer an extra kick by mixing 1 cup of powdered laundry detergent and 3 pounds of Epsom salts per 50-pound bag of lawn food. Apply the mix at half of the recommended rate with your broadcast spreader or drop spreader.

● To get rid of fairy ring on your lawn, sprinkle 2 cups of powdered laundry detergent on the area, and water well. Then mix 1 cup each of baby shampoo, antiseptic mouthwash, and ammonia in your 20 gallon hose-end sprayer, and soak the area.

# LEMONS & LEMON JUICE

## Health & Beauty

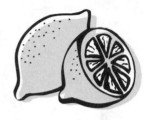

 Just can't get rid of those hiccups? Tuck a small slice of lemon under your tongue. Suck it once, hold the juice for 10 seconds, and then swallow. Your hiccups will be history.

 When you feel yourself coming down with a cold, try this old-time remedy: Fill your bathtub with water that's as hot as you can stand it. While the tub is filling, pour a jigger of rum or bourbon into a glass of hot lemonade. Then ease into the tub and drink your hot toddy. When you've finished, dry off and dive into bed. By morning, you'll be on top of the world again!

 To soothe the itch of poison ivy, insect bites, or allergies, make a paste of lemon juice and cornstarch, and rub it gently onto the problem areas.

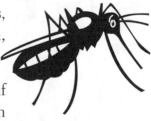

 Use lemons to help soften calluses. Rub half a lemon on your feet, elbows, and heels, and those rough spots will be smoother in no time.

 Fingernails looking dingy and tired? Clean them up with a lemon scrub. Cut a fresh, juicy lemon in half, and dig your fingers into the flesh. Keep them there for 1 minute, then rinse. Just make sure your fingers don't have cuts or scrapes on them, or you'll be in for a stinging surprise!

🍎 Here's an easy way to put blonde highlights into your hair: Combine 1 cup of lemon juice with 3 cups of brewed (and cooled) chamomile tea. Pour the solution over damp hair, then head outdoors. Sit in the sun for an hour or so, rinse thoroughly, and follow up with a good conditioner. Repeat the process until your hair reaches the desired shade of pale.

🍎 This easy routine will both tone and soften your skin: Beat 1 large egg white, then fold in the juice of half a lemon. Smooth the concoction onto your face and neck. Wait 20 minutes, and rinse it off with bottled water. Pat dry, then use a cotton ball to dab on a little witch hazel.

🍎 If you're flocked with freckles that haven't faded with age, try this old-time trick: Dissolve a pinch of sugar in 2 tablespoons of lemon juice, and dab the mixture onto each freckle with a cotton ball or tissue. Repeat the process every couple of days until the spots have lightened.

🍎 For a great facial cleanser, try this tangy recipe. First, grind lemon peels in a blender or coffee grinder. Then mix about 1 tablespoon of the grounds with enough plain yogurt to make a paste. Wash your face with the mixture, rinse with cool water, and pat dry. If your skin is on the dry side, substitute vegetable oil for the yogurt.

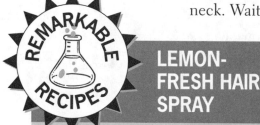

## REMARKABLE RECIPES

## LEMON-FRESH HAIR SPRAY

Tired of store-bought hair sprays? Try this super-simple alternative.

**2 cups of water**
**2 lemons**
**1 tbsp. of vodka**

Boil the water in a saucepan. While the water is boiling, peel and finely chop the lemons. Add them to the boiling water, and simmer over low heat until the lemons are soft. Cool, strain, and pour into a spray bottle. Add the vodka, and shake well. If the solution is too sticky, dilute it with a little water.

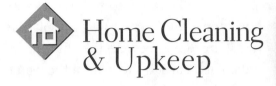

## Home Cleaning & Upkeep

◆ Make your own furniture polish by mixing 1 part lemon juice and 2 parts vegetable oil.

◆ To get scratches out of a wooden table, mix equal parts lemon juice and vegetable oil, and rub the mixture into the scratches, using a soft cotton cloth. Repeat a few times, and the scratches should disappear.

◆ To clean up spills from stovetops and ovens, mix lemon juice, water, and baking soda to make a paste. Cover the trouble spots, wait 15 minutes, and scrub the spots away.

◆ Make an all-purpose "miracle" cleaner by mixing 1 part lemon juice with 2 parts water in a spray bottle. Spray the solution on kitchen or bathroom surfaces, and wipe with a nylon-covered sponge or a mesh onion bag.

◆ Need to get ink spots out of clothes? While the ink is still wet, saturate it with lemon juice, and wash the garment in cold water with your regular detergent.

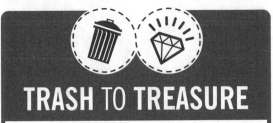

## TRASH TO TREASURE

THE OUTSIDES of citrus fruits have just as many uses as the innards. Here are three examples of how you can put those skins to work:

1. "BRUSH" YOUR TEETH: Wipe the inside of a slice of lemon or lime peel over your teeth and gums. Both fruits contain chemicals that whiten choppers *and* fight gum disease.

2. FRESHEN THE AIR: Toss a handful of your favorite citrus shavings into a pot of boiling water with cloves and cinnamon. Reduce the heat, and let the fragrant brew simmer. Or dry some slivered citrus peels and use them in your favorite potpourri recipe.

3. TRAP SLUGS AND SNAILS: Shortly before dark, set hollowed-out orange or grapefruit rinds among your plants. By morning, the skins will be filled with slimy slugs. Pick up the traps and dump them—and the pests—into a bucket of soapy water, then toss it on the compost pile.

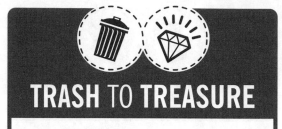

## TRASH TO TREASURE

**SOME BRANDS** of lemon juice come in plastic, lemon-shaped bottles that seem just too cute to throw away. So don't! Instead, give them one of these useful jobs:

○ **Liquid-soap dispensers in the bathroom, kitchen, or workshop**

○ **Containers to hold your homemade shampoos and hair rinses**

○ **Bathtub toys for kids**

○ **Sticky traps for insect pests (indoors or out—just coat the lemon with corn syrup or petroleum jelly, and set it in the flowerpot)**

○ **Cat toys (pry off the top, throw in a few dried beans, and put the top back on)**

◆ Did the clothes that you bleached come out with what look like rust stains? Chances are, the chlorine in the bleach caused the iron in the water to leach out. (It's a common problem in areas with hard water; rusty pipes could also be the culprit.) The solution: Saturate the stains with equal parts lemon juice and water, and wash the garments again, *without* bleach.

◆ Time to clean the silver? Mix 1 tablespoon of lemon juice, ½ cup of powdered milk, and 1½ cups of water in a bowl. Add your silver to the mix, let it sit overnight, then rinse and dry thoroughly. (If this formula doesn't make enough solution to cover your silver pieces, then double or even triple the recipe.)

◆ If you can't wait until tomorrow for sparkling silver, just pour straight lemon juice onto the piece, and polish it with a soft cotton cloth.

◆ Cutting board smelling a little fishy? Or maybe the aroma is from garlic or an onion. Whatever the scent is, banish it by wiping the board with lemon juice and rinsing with cool water.

◆ To freshen the air in your kitchen, heat the oven to 300°F, and set a whole, unpeeled lemon inside. Let it cook for about 15 minutes with the oven door slightly ajar, then turn off the oven. Let the lemon cool before you take it out.

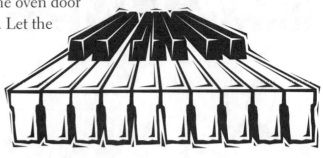

◆ Piano keys looking yellow? Dip half a lemon in salt, and tickle those ivories till they're shiny white again.

◆ Lemon juice makes dark-colored leather sparkle. Just dab a little of the juice on a soft, clean cloth, and rub it on. Finish by buffing with another soft cloth.

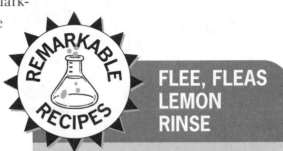

## FLEE, FLEAS LEMON RINSE

Here's a pet-pleasing rinse that will help keep felines and canines flea-free all summer long.

**1 lemon, thinly sliced**
**1 qt. of hot water**

Put the lemon slices in the water, and let the brew steep overnight. Once a day during flea season, groom your pet with a flea comb, then sponge on the lemon rinse. *Note:* Test it on a small patch of your pet's skin first—some cats and dogs are allergic to the oils in citrus fruits.

 Yard & Garden

● Repel ants, indoors or out, by putting fresh lemon slices in their pathways, or anyplace you don't want them roaming.

● Before you water potted plants, add a few drops of lemon juice to the watering can. The juice will lower the water's pH, thereby allowing the plants to take up more nutrients from the soil.

# L

# LIMES & LIME JUICE

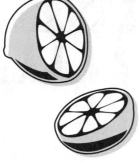

### 🍎➕ Health & Beauty

🍋 Got a headache? Cut a lime in two, and rub one half on your forehead. The throbbing will stop, pronto.

🍋 If your breath tends to be, um, less than sweet, and there's no medical or dental problem, try this remedy. At bedtime and between meals, drink the juice of one lime and a teaspoon or so of honey mixed in a glass of water.

🍋 Sore throat? Use the above recipe with a little pineapple juice added to the mix.

🍋 For healthy gums and whiter teeth, mix lime juice and salt into a paste, and rub the mixture onto your gums and teeth several times a day.

🍋 Get fish, onion, or garlic odors off of your hands by rubbing them with a slice of lime.

🍋 Tired feet? Re-energize them by massaging lime juice into the skin.

🍋 A drop of lime juice will ease the pain of a bee or fire-ant sting. (But it's *not* a substitute for medical attention. So if you have a severe reaction, get to a doctor, *now*!)

🍋 To relieve diarrhea fast, drink a cup of tea with a teaspoon or so of lime juice in it.

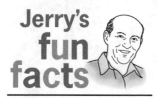

**Jerry's fun facts**

Here's something I'll bet you didn't know: Botanically speaking, limes are classified as berries. So are lemons, oranges, and pineapples!

168

🍎 Want to lighten your hair without chemicals—or a beauty-salon price tag? Just mix 1 ounce of mild shampoo with the juice of 2 limes and 1 lemon. Pour the solution onto your hair, and massage it in. Sit in the sun or under a helmet-type hair dryer for 15 to 20 minutes, then rinse.

🍎 Are you trying to quit smoking or drinking? This trick will help: Whenever you get the urge to indulge, suck on a lime. Besides curbing your desire for tobacco or alcohol, it will replace some of the vitamins, phosphates, and calcium that these substances may have drained from your system.

🍎 Are you (or other members of your family) troubled by pimples and blackheads? Wash your face with the juice of a fresh lime in a glass of boiled whole milk. If your skin is dry, add a teaspoon of glycerin to the mixture.

🍎 If tea isn't your cup of tea (see the last tip at left), try this diarrhea remedy: In a blender, purée a peeled and cored apple with about a teaspoon of lime juice, a few drops of honey, and a pinch of cinnamon. Eat it all up. (If the problem lasts more than a day or two, call your doctor.)

## REMARKABLE RECIPES

### ANTI-AGE LOTION

If age and too much time in the sun have left you with spotty skin, lighten those splotches with this tonic.

**Juice of 1 lime**
**Juice of 1 lemon**
**4 tbsp. of plain yogurt**
**2 tbsp. of honey**

Mix all of the ingredients together, and gently massage the lotion into each spot at least once a week. Store the mixture in a covered container in the refrigerator.

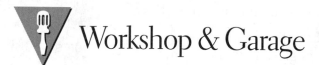

## Home Cleaning & Upkeep

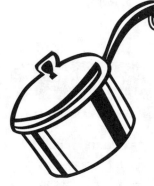

◆ Nothing beats lime juice for getting stubborn dirt out of clothes. Just saturate the spot, rub in a pinch (or a few drops) of your regular detergent, and launder as you usually would.

◆ Clean copper or brass by cutting a lime in half, dipping it in salt, and rubbing the metal. Rinse with cold water.

◆ Get "rainbow" marks off stainless steel pots by rubbing the stains with a cut lime.

◆ If a stained pot is made of aluminum or enamel, fill the pan with water, add a cut lime, and boil until the stains disappear. Use half the fruit for a small pot, or both halves for a larger one.

## Workshop & Garage

▼ Clean your car's chrome by rubbing it with lime juice on a soft cotton cloth.

▼ Has someone been smoking in your car? Clean the film off the windows by washing them with a solution of 2 tablespoons of lime juice and 1 quart of water.

▼ When you're painting outdoors, add a few drops of lime juice to the paint to keep insects away from all the action.

# LIP BALM

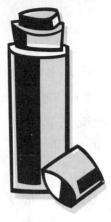

 ## Health & Beauty

 Cut yourself shaving? Stop the bleeding with a dab of lip balm.

 To protect your skin from windburn, rub some lip balm on your face *before* you hit the ski slopes, sledding trail, or outdoor ice rink.

 When a ring just won't slide off your finger, coat the skin under and around the ring with lip balm.

 Are your eyebrow hairs a little bushier than you'd like? Smooth them down with lip balm. (It'll keep the ends of a fly-away mustache under control, too!)

 Before you dye your hair, wipe lip balm along your hairline. That way, you'll color your hair and *not* your skin.

 Moisturize dry cuticles by rubbing some lip balm on them. Massage the balm all around each nailbed, then gently push back cuticles.

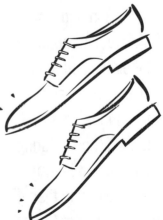

## Home Cleaning & Upkeep

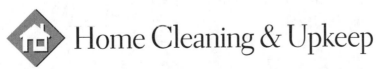

 When you need a shoeshine in a hurry and you're out of polish, rub the leather with lip balm, and buff with a clean, soft cloth.

171

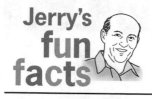
◆ Tired of struggling with a stubborn zipper? It'll run smoothly if you lubricate the teeth with a little lip balm.

◆ Drawers and windows will open and close more easily if you smear the gliders with lip balm.

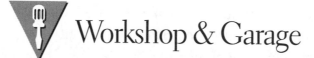

# Workshop & Garage

▼ To keep car battery terminals from corroding, rub them with lip balm.

▼ Wipe nails and screws with lip balm so they'll go into wood more easily.

▼ Got tiny rust specks on your tools? Stop those little spots from turning into big ones by washing and drying the tools, then dabbing them with lip balm.

▼ When a hand tool's moving parts are sluggish and you're fresh out of lubricating oil, rub a little lip balm over the pieces instead.

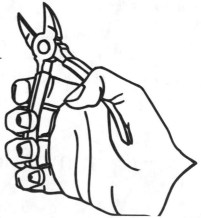

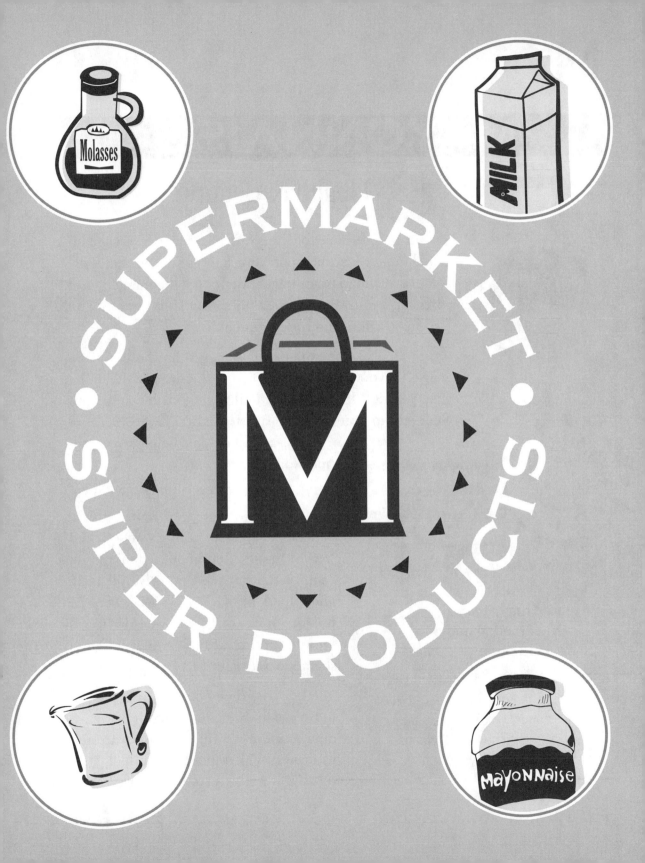

# M

# MAYONNAISE

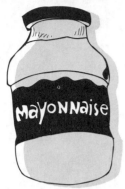

## Health & Beauty

👆 Plain old mayonnaise makes a great hair conditioner. Just shampoo your hair as you normally do, towel dry, and massage regular mayo (*not* the miracle salad dressing!) into your hair. Let it sit for 15 minutes or so, shampoo again, and rinse thoroughly.

👆 For extra-dry or damaged hair, use mayonnaise as you would a hot-oil treatment. Just heat the mayo until it's warm (don't boil it!), and rub it into your hair. Wrap your head in a warm towel, wait 15 to 30 minutes, and shampoo with warm (not hot) water.

👆 Here's an alternative treatment for dry or damaged hair. Purée a banana in a blender until it's smooth and free of lumps. Add about 1 tablespoon each of mayonnaise and olive oil to it, and blend until creamy. Massage the mixture into your hair, wait 15 to 30 minutes, rinse with warm water, and shampoo as usual.

👆 Use mayonnaise to remove eye makeup. Just smooth the mayo onto your eyelids with your fingertip, and wipe away with a moist cotton ball. (Just be careful not to get any *in* your eyes!)

## REMARKABLE RECIPES

### HOMEMADE COLD CREAM

This triple-treat recipe will remove makeup, and clean and soften your skin.

**½ cup of mayonnaise**
**1 tbsp. of melted butter**
**Juice of 1 lemon or 1 lime**

Mix all of the ingredients together, and store the cream in the refrigerator in a tightly closed glass jar. Use it as you would any facial cleanser, and rinse with cold water.

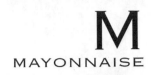

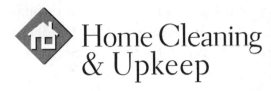

## Home Cleaning & Upkeep

◆ To get tar out of clothing, slather mayonnaise on the spots, let it soak into the fabric, and launder or dry-clean the garment as usual.

◆ When you find crayon marks on wooden furniture, rub on some mayo, let it sit for a minute or so, and wipe clean with a damp cloth.

◆ Remove white rings from tabletops by rubbing them with a little mayonnaise on a soft cloth. Immediately wipe off the excess.

◆ Make a polish for wooden floors or furniture by mixing 2 parts mayonnaise with 1 part lemon juice. Apply with a soft cloth or sponge mop, and buff with a clean cloth.

## Kids & Pets

■ Has chewing gum found its way into your child's hair? Massage mayonnaise into the glob, leave it for 5 minutes or so, then comb it out.

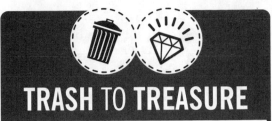

## TRASH TO TREASURE

**MAYONNAISE JARS,** with those tight-fitting, screw-on plastic lids, are some of the handiest helpers you could ask for—indoors or out. What's more, they come in a whole range of sizes from mini to gigantic, so you can choose the one that suits the task at hand. Here's just a sampling of their talents:

○ Canisters for all sorts of dry goods, such as pasta, flour, and crackers

○ Storage jars for leftovers

○ Organizers for your sewing space, office, craft area, or workshop

○ Containers for homemade cleaners, lotions, and pest-control tonics

○ Holders for bathroom gear, such as cotton balls, first-aid supplies, and small cosmetics like lipstick and eye makeup

○ Traps for flying insect pests

And don't forget the lids! They're just the ticket for dishing up the last supper for ants, roaches, mice, and other small, pesky pests in the yard.

# M
## MAYONNAISE

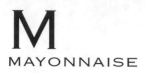
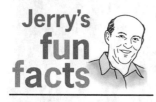
■ When Fido or Fluffy takes a run through the brambles and comes home wearing a bunch of them, massage mayonnaise into your pet's fur. The stickers will comb right out.

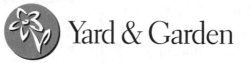

# Workshop & Garage

▼ Mayonnaise will get grease, tar, or pine pitch off your car, your tools, or just about anything else. Just rub on the mayo, let it sit for a few minutes, and wipe it off.

▼ To keep wooden tool handles smooth, clean, and free of cracks, rub them every now and again with a mixture of 2 parts mayonnaise to 1 part lemon juice on a soft cloth.

# Yard & Garden

● Use mayonnaise to make your houseplants clean and shiny. How? Just mix the mayo with enough water to form a thick paste, apply it to the leaves with a soft cloth, and wipe off any excess.

● When it's time to put your garden tools away for the winter, keep them rust-free with mayonnaise. Just wash the tools, dry them, and rub mayo onto all the metal parts, using a soft cloth. Rub off any excess before stashing the tools.

# MILK & CREAM

 Health & Beauty

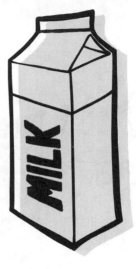

🍎 Got pepper in your eye? Flush it out with a few drops of milk.

🍎 To ease the pain of sunburn, poison ivy, or hot-pepper burns, dip a soft cloth in milk, and gently wash the affected skin.

🍎 Soothe rough, red hands by rubbing a little warm milk into your skin each night.

🍎 Are your eyes swollen, tired, or irritated (maybe from too many hours in front of the computer)? Soak two cotton pads in ice-cold cream or whole milk. Lie down in a comfortable place, put one pad over each eye, and relax for 10 minutes or so. Rinse with warm water, then cool water. The fat content of the liquid will soothe and moisturize the delicate skin around your eyes.

🍎 Need a fast, simple eye-makeup remover? Just dampen a cotton ball with heavy cream, and gently wipe your lids.

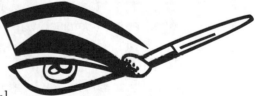

🍎 For a quick and easy facial cleanser, mix 2 tablespoons of whole milk with 2 tablespoons of warm (not hot) honey. Rinse your face with water, massage the cleanser in for a couple of minutes, rinse it off, and pat your face dry. This mixture doesn't keep well, so make it as you need it.

When you're tired and irritated, try this simple soother: In a blender, mix 2 cups of powdered milk (dry), 1 cup of cornstarch, and (if you like) your favorite scented oil. Add ½ cup of the mixture to hot bath water, sink into the tub, and relax. Store the remaining mixture in an airtight container at room temperature.

Here's how to make a peach of a moisturizer: Peel a large, ripe peach. Mash it through a sieve to get as much juice as possible. Mix the peach juice with an equal amount of fresh cream, and massage a small amount of the mixture into your skin. Store the remainder in the refrigerator in an airtight container, and use it within a week.

## REMARKABLE RECIPES

### LEMON FACE CREAM

Use this cream every night to keep your skin satiny soft.

**1 lemon**
**¼ cup or so of heavy cream (whipping cream)**
**Piece of muslin or other light cloth**

From the center of the lemon, cut a slice that's about ¼ inch thick. Lay it flat in a clean glass jar that has a lid. Pour in enough cream to cover the lemon slice, cover the container with the cloth, and let it sit at room temperature for 24 hours, or until it's about the thickness of face cream. Replace the cloth with the regular jar lid, and put it in the refrigerator. Rub the cream into your skin every night at bedtime. The mixture will eventually spoil, so make a new batch every week.

## Home Cleaning & Upkeep

◆ To keep leather upholstery soft and prevent it from cracking, wipe it with milk, then use a clean, soft cloth to polish it. Do this several times a year. (This also works well for leather car upholstery.)

◆ Shine up leather shoes and purses by rubbing them with a soft cloth dipped in milk.

◆ Clean concrete walkways or patios this way: Make a half-and-half solution of whole milk and regular cola (not diet), pour the mix on the dirty surface, and scrub with a stiff brush. Rinse with the garden hose.

◆ To make a linoleum floor sparkle, pour a little skim milk on it, and spread the milk around with a mop. Wipe away any excess from cracks and crevices, and follow this up with a warm-water rinse.

◆ Use milk to banish ballpoint pen ink from cotton and synthetic fabrics. Dampen a sponge with the milk, dab the stain until it's gone, and launder as usual. (Be patient, though; it may take a while to get all of the ink out.)

◆ To get fruit or wine stains off of clothes or table linens, pour salt on the spots, and soak the fabric in milk until the marks vanish.

◆ Get silver clean and shiny with milk. Put the pieces in a container, and sprinkle them with a mixture of equal parts of salt and cream of tartar. Pour in enough milk to cover the silver, let it soak for 2 to 3 hours, take it out, and polish with a soft cloth.

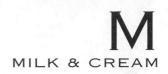

## TRASH TO TREASURE

WHETHER YOU buy milk and cream by the pint, the quart, or the half-gallon, those wax-paper containers are worth their weight in moo-juice. In the garden, they're perfect for starting seeds and protecting young plants from grubs and cutworms (just slice off the top and bottom, and push them into the soil around your seedlings). Here are two more ways to say "Carry on, cartons!"

1. Fill them up with water, and put them in the freezer. They'll take up space, which will make the freezer run more efficiently. Plus, when a heat wave strikes, you can take out a carton, set it in front of a fan, and presto—an instant air conditioner!

2. Turn them into building blocks for your kids or grandkids. For each block, you'll need two cartons of the same size. Cut off the tops, wash the containers thoroughly, and let them dry. Shove one carton inside the other, open ends first, and you're good to go.

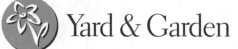

# Yard & Garden

● To protect plants against viruses, mix 2 tablespoons of milk in 1 gallon of water. Pour the solution into a hand-held spray bottle, and spray the foliage every two or three weeks throughout the growing season.

● Repel whiteflies by misting your plants with a mixture of 1 cup of sour milk, 2 tablespoons of flour, and 1 quart of warm water. (To make sour milk, put 1 tablespoon of vinegar in a measuring cup, and pour in fresh milk to the 1-cup line.)

● Feed your outdoor ferns by spraying them to the point of runoff with a mixture of 1 cup of milk and 1 tablespoon of Epsom salts in a 20 gallon hose-end sprayer.

● Keep leftover seeds fresh by storing them in powdered milk. Put 1 part seeds to 1 part powdered milk in a glass jar with a tight-fitting lid, and put it in the refrigerator (not the freezer).

● Head off cutworm problems by trapping the egg-laying moths with this trick: Fill a wide, flat pan with milk, and set it in the garden. Beside it, place a lighted lantern so that it shines on the milk. The moths will zero in on the glowing target, fall into the milk, and drown.

## REMARKABLE RECIPES

### TIMELY TOMATO TONIC

This powerful powder will help your tomato plants fend off nasty diseases.

**3 cups of compost**
**½ cup of Epsom salts**
**1 tbsp. of baking soda**
**½ cup of powdered nonfat milk**

Combine the first three ingredients in a bucket, and add a handful of the mix to the planting hole. After planting, sprinkle a little of the powdered milk on top of the soil. Repeat every few weeks during the growing season.

# MOLASSES

 ## Health & Beauty

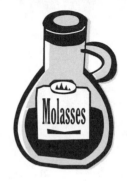

Want to make your fingernails and toenails harder and stronger? Eat plenty of molasses. It's rich in sulfur—one of the keys to maintaining healthy nails.

Soften and deep-clean your skin with this facial masque: In a blender, mix half an avocado, 2 tablespoons of orange juice, and 1 teaspoon each of molasses and honey. Smooth the mixture onto your skin, wait 30 to 40 minutes, and remove the masque, using a damp, warm washcloth. Store any extra in a covered container in the refrigerator; it will keep for two or three days.

Troubled by varicose veins? Make them fade by eating 2 to 3 teaspoons of blackstrap molasses daily. It will improve your circulation, thus opening up the channels and clearing up the discoloration.

Here's a handy tip if you (or someone you know) are in the second half of a pregnancy and are suffering leg aches and muscle cramps: Every day, drink 1 cup of hot water with 1 teaspoon of blackstrap molasses dissolved in it. It's rich in calcium and magnesium, which help stave off those awful aches and pains.

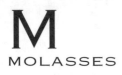

# Home Cleaning & Upkeep

◆ Got grass stains on your clothes or white sneakers? Rub molasses into the spots, let the garments sit overnight, and wash them with mild soap (not detergent). The stains will vanish like magic.

◆ Your Christmas tree will keep its needles longer if you follow this routine: When you bring the tree home, cut 1 or 2 inches off the bottom of the trunk, and immediately set it into a bucket of cold water with 1 cup of molasses added to it. Let the tree soak for two or three days before you move it to its stand and start trimming it.

◆ Need dark corn syrup for a recipe, and you're fresh out? No problem: For every cup of dark syrup that you want, substitute ¾ cup of light corn syrup and ¼ cup of molasses.

## REMARKABLE RECIPES

### ENERGIZING ELIXIR

Long before sports drinks came on the market, folks took a break from hard work or play by sitting under a shady tree and drinking this restorative beverage.

**2 ½ cups of sugar**
**1 cup of dark molasses**
**½ cup of vinegar (either white or cider)**
**1 gal. of water**

Mix all of the ingredients together in a big jug. Then get your team out of the sun, and pour everyone a nice, tall, refreshing glass.

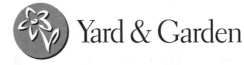

# Yard & Garden

● To make a potent ant killer, mix 2 parts molasses, 1 part sugar, and 1 part dry yeast powder. Spoon a little of the goo onto pieces of paper, and set them around the problem area.

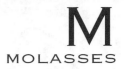

● Grasshoppers on the rampage? Bury a jar up to its rim and fill it with a mixture of equal parts molasses and water. The 'hoppers will dive right in, and they won't get out.

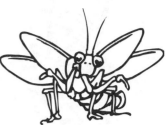

● Fly troubles will be a thing of the past if you beat an egg yolk with 1 tablespoon of molasses and a pinch of black pepper, and serve up the concoction in shallow cans or jar lids. The flies will dive in for a three-point landing, and they won't take off again.

● Say goodbye to moles by pouring molasses into their runs. It gums up their fur and sends them off in search of less sticky quarters. (If you want, you can add just a little water to make the molasses easier to handle.)

● Use molasses as a good all-purpose, organic fertilizer. Apply it at a rate of 4 or 5 tablespoons per gallon of water.

● Jump-start your compost pile by sprinkling it with a half-and-half mix of molasses and water. Molasses increases microbial activity, helping the organic matter break down faster. Water makes the molasses easier to handle.

● Are nematodes running roughshod through your soil? This simple technique will polish them off: Combine 1 cup of molasses and 1 can of beer in your 20 gallon hose-end sprayer, and thoroughly soak the problem area.

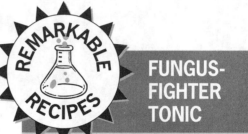

**REMARKABLE RECIPES**

## FUNGUS-FIGHTER TONIC

This terrific tonic works like magic to fend off foul fungi on ornamental or edible plants.

**½ cup of molasses**
**½ cup of powdered milk**
**1 tsp. of baking soda**
**1 gal. of warm water**

Mix the molasses, powdered milk, and baking soda into a paste. Place the mixture into an old pantyhose leg, and let it steep in the warm water for several hours. Strain, pour the remaining liquid into a hand-held spray bottle, and spritz your fungus-prone plants every week or so during the growing season.

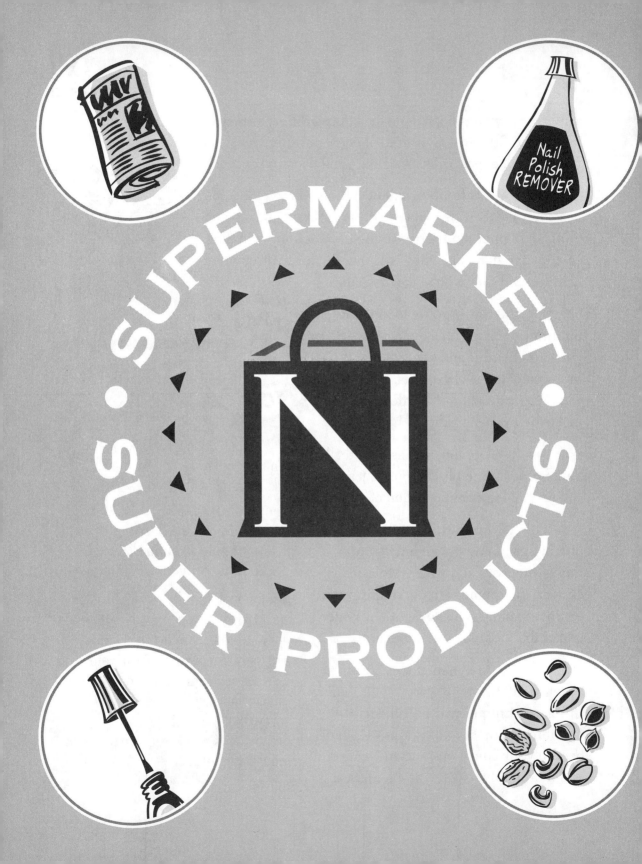

# NAIL POLISH

 ## Health & Beauty

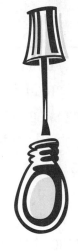

When you bring a new prescription home from the drugstore, paint over the label with clear nail polish. That way, even if the bottle gets wet, the ink won't run and you'll still be able to read the instructions.

Do you have trouble lining up those all-but-invisible arrows on childproof medicine bottles? Paint the marks with brightly colored nail polish, and you'll get 'em together on the first try, every time.

Brush clear nail polish onto the bottom edges of metal shaving-cream and hair-spray cans to keep them from rusting.

Got a screw that keeps popping out of your eyeglasses? Put a dab of clear nail polish on top of it, and the little thing will stay put.

## Home Cleaning & Upkeep

If you drip-dry clothes on wire hangers, nicks or rust spots on the hangers can end up staining your clothes. Keep 'em sealed with clear nail polish.

Are your shoelaces fraying at the ends? Twist the strands together tightly, dampen them just a little, dip them in clear nail polish, and let them dry.

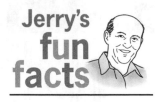

Like many other common products, including spaghetti, nail polish originated in China. By about 3,000 B.C., the Chinese were making the stuff by combining egg white, gelatin, gum arabic, and beeswax. The art of nail care goes back a long way in other regions, too. In southern Babylonia, archeologists found a solid gold manicure set that they reckoned was at least 4,000 years old!

◆ After you've dyed a pair of shoes, coat the heels with clear nail polish to keep the new color from coming off.

◆ Stop pantyhose and stocking runs from spreading by dabbing them with clear nail polish.

◆ Paint clear nail polish onto costume jewelry to help it hold its shine and color.

◆ Are your stereo speakers rattling? Take off the covers and examine the cones inside. Chances are one of them has a small tear in the fabric—and you can make it sound like new again by sealing it with a spot of nail polish.

◆ Does your skin break out in a rash every time you wear your wristwatch? Solve the problem by coating the underside of the watch with clear nail polish. (Use this same trick for any metal jewelry that causes a reaction.)

◆ Keep belt buckles and metal buttons shiny by painting them with clear nail polish. For best results, apply four coats, letting each coat dry before brushing on the next one.

◆ Got a hem or an inner seam that's starting to open? Brush on some clear nail polish to hold the fabric in place until you can sew it back together.

◆ Make buttons stay on longer by dabbing the button thread with clear nail polish.

◆ Fresh out of glue? Use clear nail polish instead. It's perfect for holding lightweight fabric, plastic, or paper (such as stamps that you've taken off of envelopes).

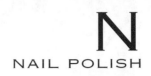

◆ Threading a needle is a snap if you dip the end of the thread in clear nail polish before you poke it through the eye of the needle. (Just make sure you let the polish dry first.)

◆ Do your measuring cups have faded gradation marks that you can hardly see? Repaint the lines with brightly colored nail polish.

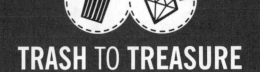

## TRASH TO TREASURE

**WHENEVER YOU empty a bottle of nail polish, wash the bottle and the little brush thoroughly (with help from nail polish remover), and tuck it away. Then, the next time you paint a room or a piece of furniture, pour some of the paint into the bottle. It'll come in mighty handy for touching up dings and scratches down the road!**

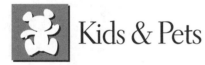 Kids & Pets

■ When your favorite young artist or writer presents you with a small sample of his work, protect it for posterity with a coat of clear nail polish.

■ Would you like to give a photo or drawing a textured finish? Try this trick: Pour clear nail polish into a shallow dish, dip a 1-inch-wide paintbrush into it, and paint the surface of the picture. (Be sure to practice on something you don't care about *before* you try your hand on a family treasure!)

■ Do you ever take the kids to fairs and other events where they stamp your hand for re-entry? To keep the mark from fading before its time, cover it with clear nail polish.

■ If you have trouble seeing the raised gradation marks on plastic baby bottles, dab the lines with brightly colored nail polish.

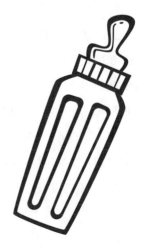

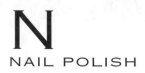

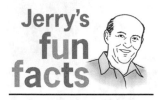

Nowadays, you can wear any color nail polish you want, and there are hundreds of colors to choose from. But that hasn't always been the case. In ancient Egypt, for instance, a woman's nail color indicated her social rank. Commoners could wear pale tones, while red was reserved for royal fingers. Queen Nefertiti favored ruby, while Cleopatra went in for a deep, rusty red.

■ Does your child or grandchild have a favorite toy that she takes to preschool or daycare? Paint her name on the bottom of the toy with nail polish. That way, it's less likely to be taken.

■ Are there small children around your house who can't tell the hot water faucets from the cold ones? Protect those tiny fingers from burns by marking the hot faucets with red nail polish—and, of course, make sure the youngsters know those marks mean "Don't touch!"

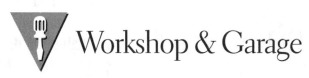

# Workshop & Garage

▼ Here's a great—though *temporary*—solution for that sad moment when you discover a scratch on your car door. Wipe the scratch with soapy water, rinse and dry it well, and give it a coat or two of clear nail polish. It will keep the scratch clean and rust-free until you can take your chariot to a body shop.

▼ Has a flying stone left a small dent in your car's windshield? Drip a little clear nail polish into the hole, let it dry, and add a few more drops. Repeat the procedure until you've filled the hole.

▼ Coat the heads of nails and screws with clear polish to prevent rust.

▼ Got drawer pulls that keep coming loose? Take out the screws, dip them in nail polish, and replace them. They'll hold tight now!

# NAIL POLISH REMOVER

## Home Cleaning & Upkeep

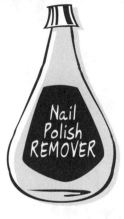

◆ Get rid of scuff marks on a linoleum floor by wiping them with nail polish remover. (Test this method on a hidden part of the floor first.)

◆ To remove scuffs and grease stains from patent leather shoes, gently rub the spots with nail polish remover. Don't rub too hard, though, or you could take the finish off along with the dirt!

◆ Spilled ink on your best cotton shirt? Saturate the stains with nail polish remover, and blot dry with a clean cloth. Repeat if necessary, and launder as usual.

◆ Repair burns on a wooden table this way: First, swab the spot with nail polish remover, and scrape gently with a dull knife until the black crust is gone. Fill the indentation with clear nail polish, one thin layer at a time, letting it dry between coats. Finish with a coat of your regular furniture polish.

◆ Remove minor scratches from watch faces and any other hard plastic surfaces by dipping a cotton ball in nail polish remover, and rubbing gently until the marks fade away.

◆ When you find some great-looking brass candlesticks at a tag sale, don't pass them up because the lacquer finish is damaged. Strip the old coating by rubbing it with nail polish remover on a soft cloth. Then either polish the brass, or have it professionally relacquered.

# Workshop & Garage

▼ Got an old decal that's clinging for dear life to your car's window? Soak that picture with nail polish remover for a few minutes, and scrape it away with a razor blade.

▼ Nail polish remover can make bumper-sticker removal a snap, too. Saturate the sticker, and ease it off with a razor blade or sharp scraper.

▼ Clean pliers, tin snips, and other cutting tools with a little nail polish remover.

▼ Did your latest project leave you with superglue all over your hands? Get it off by soaking a cotton pad or cloth in nail polish remover and holding it on your skin until the glue disappears. Just don't pick at the glue or try to peel it off.

## TRASH TO TREASURE

**PLASTIC TUBS** from ice cream, margarine, and other soft foods are trash-to-treasure goldmines. There's just one drawback: They come with writing all over them, and you might not want that on your (let's say) craft-supply containers. So what do you do? Reach for some nail polish remover. Just rub it onto the lid or the body of the tub, and wipe the ink right off.

# NEWSPAPER

##  Home Cleaning & Upkeep

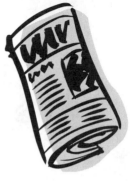

◆ To get grease or dampness out of metal garbage cans, burn crumpled-up newspaper inside them. (Just be sure to leave the lid off!)

◆ The next time you get caught in a storm and come home with soaking wet shoes, follow this routine: Stuff the shoes with newspaper, and lay them on their sides to dry, away from any heat source.

◆ Fresh out of firewood? Don't run to the store for fake logs. Make a supply from newspaper instead. Roll two or three papers tightly together, and wrap them with wire or twine. Then light your fire, baby!

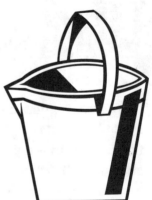

◆ Got a plastic bucket or garbage pail that's smelling pretty rank? Fill the container with black and white newspaper, cover it, and let it sit overnight. By morning, the odor will be gone.

## 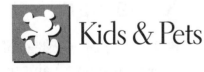 Kids & Pets

■ Spray the newspaper comics section with hair spray, and use it as gift wrap for a child's (or a young-at-heart grownup's) present.

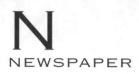
■ Here's a clever idea for a new-baby gift: Wrap it in the front page of the newspaper from the day the child was born. Or use the birth-announcements page, and draw a big, colorful star around the "star's" vital statistics. Either way, be sure to coat the paper with hair spray before you wrap your package.

■ Use hair-sprayed comics to cover lidded cardboard boxes (like the ones that photocopy paper comes in), and use them to store toys and out-of-season clothes in a child's room.

■ Making Halloween costumes for the kids? Cut the patterns out of newspaper.

■ Fresh out of cat litter? Run some newspaper through a paper shredder, and use it instead. Or line your cat's litter box with newspaper to absorb odors and make your regular litter last a bit longer.

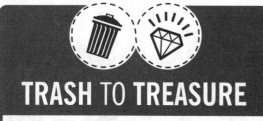

## TRASH TO TREASURE

USING OLD newspapers to wash windows is a classic trash-to-treasure tip. But times—and *The Times*—are changing. Nowadays, many newspapers are printed with soy-based inks, which don't do as good a job on glass as the old chemical-based inks did. On the positive side, the new inks are much less toxic, which makes them better for garden-variety work like making compost (shred the paper first), or wrapping around green tomatoes to make them ripen well.

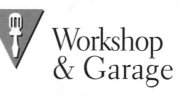

# Workshop & Garage

▼ Use newspaper instead of masking tape when you're painting around windows. Just dampen a straight edge of the paper, and press it onto the glass next to the wood. When the paper dries, peel it off.

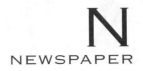

▼ If you have tools that you don't use very often, treat them the same way you would off-duty gardening gear: Give them a light coat of oil (any kind will do), and wrap them in newspaper to keep them clean and rust-free.

▼ In winter, keep a stack of newspapers in the trunk of your car. If you get stuck in ice or snow, shove a few thicknesses under your rear wheels (or front, if you have a front-wheel-drive vehicle). The paper will give you the traction you need to get going.

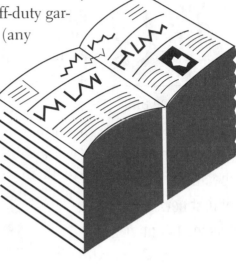

## Yard & Garden

● Make seed-starting pots using newspaper and a soda can. For each pot, cut a strip of paper that's about a foot long and 6 inches wide. Wrap the paper around the soda can lengthwise, with about 2 inches hanging over the bottom. Fold the extra piece up to the base of the can, press it in place with your fingers, and remove the can. Add seed-starting mix and pack the pots tightly into a flat that has drainage holes.

● Blanch leeks, celery, cauliflower, and chard (that is, make them mature to white or light green in the garden) by wrapping the base of the plants with newspaper, and tying it shut with twine. Keep the newspaper on the plant until it's ready to harvest.

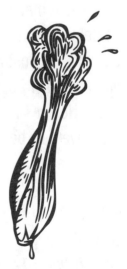

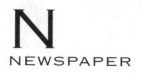

## Jerry's fun facts

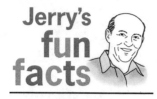

Richard Pierce and Benjamin Harris were the printer and editor, respectively, of the very first newspaper published in America. It had the straightforward title of *Publick Occurrences, Both Foreign and Domestick,* and it made its debut—and its closing—in Boston on September 25, 1690. Nearly 14 years went by before John Campbell launched the Colonies' first successful paper, the *Boston News-Letter,* on April 24, 1704.

● Toss torn, shredded, or chopped-up newspaper onto your compost pile. It helps balance the high-nitrogen "green" ingredients, such as grass clippings or kitchen scraps. Plus, it attracts lots of earthworms, who will quickly turn all that organic matter into "black gold."

● Going on a brief vacation, and no one's on hand to water your houseplants? This trick will save the day: Line the bottom of your bathtub with newspapers, and soak them with water. Set the plants on top of the wet papers, and they'll stay moist and happy for at least two weeks.

● Trap earwigs by setting out sections of dampened, rolled-up newspaper in your garden at night. The next morning, the rolls will be filled with the tiny bugs seeking shelter. Stomp on them, or drown them in soapy water to finish them off.

● If you're growing tomatoes this summer, keep their roots moist and happy by tucking some wadded-up newspaper in the bottom of each planting hole. As water leaches through the soil, the paper will absorb and hold it—right where the roots can tap into the supply through the long, hot summer.

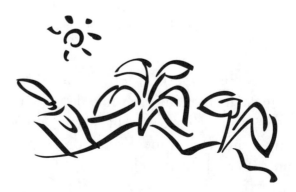

# NUTS

 Health & Beauty

For a super-simple cleanser, you can't beat this: Grind shelled almonds to a fine powder in a blender or coffee grinder. Wet your face, rub the almond powder into your skin, and rinse.

This facial scrub will keep your skin soft and squeaky clean: Grind 2 tablespoons of almond slivers in a blender or coffee grinder, and mix the resulting powder with 2 teaspoons of milk, ½ teaspoon of flour, and enough honey to make a thick paste. Rub it into your skin, and rinse with warm water.

Try this pore-tightening facial masque to get your skin glowing: Combine ½ cup of dry oatmeal, 1 tablespoon each of honey and cider vinegar, and 1 teaspoon of ground almonds. Moisten your face with a warm washcloth, and smooth on the mixture, avoiding the eye area. Wait until the masque dries (about 20 minutes) and remove it with a warm, damp washcloth. Rinse your face with warm water, and gently pat dry.

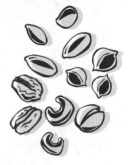

**ALMOND FACE CLEANSER**

Here's a facial cleanser that's perfect for all skin types, and you can put it together in a flash.

**1 cup of shelled almonds**
**1 cup of dry oatmeal**
**1 cup of dried orange peel**

Put all of the ingredients in a blender or food processor, and chop until they form a fine powder. Scoop some into the palm of your hand, add a few drops of water, and rub it onto your face. (Be careful not to get any in your eyes.) Rinse with warm water, and pat dry. Store the powder in an airtight container at room temperature.

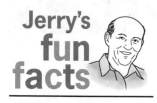

Here are some things you may not know about almonds:

• They are the oldest, most widely grown, and most extensively used nuts in the world.

• They are one of two nuts mentioned in the Bible (pistachio is the other).

• Almonds were brought to the New World by Spanish missionaries to California.

• They have more calcium and fiber than any other nut or seed — so eat 'em up!

 If you want to keep your heart healthy, I say nuts to you! Studies at major medical schools have shown that eating a handful of nuts (especially walnuts, pecans, and almonds) five or more times a week cuts your heart attack risk in half compared with folks who never eat them.

## Home Cleaning & Upkeep

◆ To remove scratches from dark wood furniture, floors, or woodwork, reach for some nuts. Brazil nuts, pecans, or black walnuts work best. Simply shell the nuts and rub the nutmeat directly into the scratch, being careful to keep it away from surrounding areas (so as not to darken them inadvertently).

◆ When you're cooking cabbage, get rid of that distinctive aroma by tossing a whole, unshelled walnut into the water.

◆ Make fabric dye, wood stain, or ink from black-walnut hulls. There are many ways to do this, but here's the ultra-easy method: Put 1 or 2 cups of walnuts (in the shells) into a Crock-Pot®, and add just enough water to cover them. Cook all night on low heat. In the morning, the water will be a rich brown color. Strain out the nuts, and you're good to go!

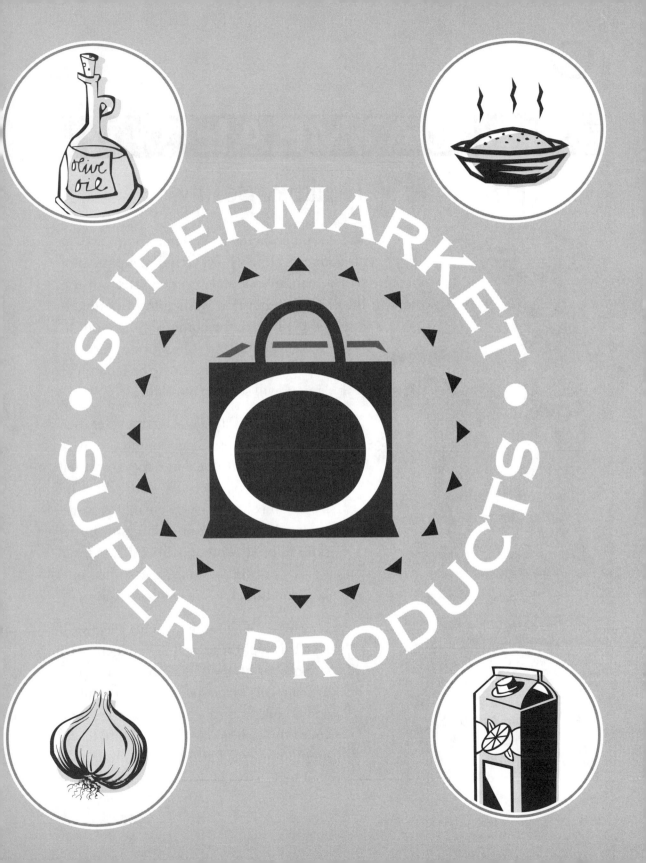

SUPERMARKET · SUPER PRODUCTS ·

# OATMEAL

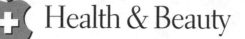 Health & Beauty

 Are you bothered by eczema? Stop the pain and itch with oatmeal. Here's how: Grind a cup or so of dry oatmeal in a blender or coffee grinder, and put the powder in the center of a cotton washcloth or handkerchief. Gather up the corners of the cloth to make a pouch, dip it in warm water, and dab it onto the eczema. The oatmeal "juice" will soothe your skin.

 Here's a terrific cleanser for all skin types: Grind about ¼ cup of old-fashioned oatmeal in a coffee grinder until it's the consistency of coarse flour. In a bowl, mix it with heavy cream to form a paste. (If you have oily skin, substitute skim milk.) Let the mixture thicken for a minute or two, then massage it into your face and throat. Rinse with cool water.

 Your tired, aching feet will love this nighttime treat: Mix together ¼ cup of coarsely ground almonds, ¼ cup of dry oatmeal, 3 tablespoons of cocoa butter, and 2 tablespoons of honey. Massage into your skin, pull on cotton socks, and leave them on overnight. In the morning, rinse your tootsies with cool water.

**REMARKABLE RECIPES**

## OATMEAL SCRUB

This bathtime treat cleanses, tones, and softens your skin all over.

**1 cup of dry oatmeal**
**½ cup of almonds, coarsely ground**
**1 ripe avocado, peeled and mashed**

Mix the oatmeal and almonds, and put the mixture in a bath mitt or a clean pantyhose foot. Peel the avocado, and mash it in a small bowl. When you're in the tub or shower, use the filled mitt to scoop up some avocado, and rub it onto your skin. After your bath, rinse, pat dry, and follow up with your regular moisturizer.

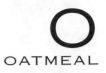
For a gentle, exfoliating face and body scrub, mix 1 part dry oatmeal and 1 part baking soda with 3 parts water. Apply to your face in a circular motion, or use it to scrub rough elbows and knees.

# Yard & Garden

Here's a great food for any flowering plant: Combine equal parts of dry oatmeal, human hair, and crushed, dry dog chow. Mix a handful of it into the soil every two to three weeks during the growing season. (You can ask your hair stylist or barber for discarded hair cuttings.)

To get outdoor container plants off to a great start, use this variation: Mix 2 cups each of dry oatmeal and crushed dry dog food, a pinch of human hair, and 1½ teaspoons of sugar. Add 2 tablespoons of this mix to moistened, professional potting soil.

When you divide your perennials, add a handful of dry oatmeal to the soil mix before replanting each division.

## TRASH TO TREASURE

AS WE all know, you should eat plenty of fiber-rich oatmeal for a healthy heart—and use it to soften your face, soothe your aching feet, and nourish your plants. That means you wind up with a *lot* of empty oatmeal canisters. What can you do with them? Plenty! Here's a roundup:

○ Storage containers for the workshop, garage, or any room in the house

○ Holders for paintbrushes, sculpting tools, or screwdrivers

○ Molds for big pillar candles

○ Soap molds (slice the soap into individual, round bars after it's hardened)

○ Gift boxes

○ Building blocks or bongo drums for the kids

○ "Vases" for dried flowers or herbs

  (For some of these ideas, you'll want to cover the container in decorative paper or fabric; for others, just leave the kindly Quaker gentleman in place.)

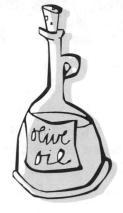

# OLIVE OIL

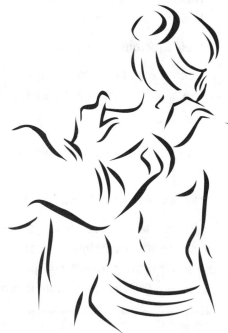

## Health & Beauty

Looking for the perfect skin moisturizer? Look no further—reach for virgin olive oil for super-soft skin.

For a soothing, moisturizing bath, heat a few tablespoons of olive oil, and rub the warm oil on your skin. Wait 5 minutes, then ease into the tub, and lather up.

The next time you take a bath, treat your feet to this moisturizing salt rub. Moisten a handful of Epsom salts with a small amount of olive oil. Then scrub your feet until the salts have dissolved and the oil has softened up your skin.

Got a scar that won't go away? Massage a little olive oil into it every day. Over time, it will lighten the scar and reduce the raised, "proud" flesh.

Relieve your bursitis by massaging olive oil into your shoulder or upper arm once a day.

Relieve an earache by inserting a few drops of olive oil into the affected ear and plugging it with cotton. Then lie down with the sore ear on a hot water bottle or heating pad.

🍎 Here's an old-fashioned cough remedy that works like a charm: Mix 3 to 4 tablespoons of lemon juice, 1 cup of honey, and ½ cup of olive oil. Heat for 5 minutes (don't boil), and stir vigorously for 2 minutes. Take 1 teaspoon every 2 hours.

🍎 Fresh out of shaving cream? Slather on some olive oil instead. (Ladies—this will make shaved legs sleek and smooth.)

🍎 Is your hair starting to fall out? The old-timers in my family swore by this treatment: Once or twice a week, beat a raw egg with about 1 tablespoon of olive oil, massage it into your hair and scalp, and leave it in place for a few minutes. Then rinse it out with warm water. (But I'm *not* guaranteeing this as a cure for baldness!)

🍎 When a jellyfish or man-of-war takes the fun out of your swim, apply olive oil to the sting site, and seek medical attention immediately.

🍎 Treat a case of constipation by taking 1 to 3 tablespoons of olive oil. If this mild laxative doesn't do the trick in a few days, see your doctor.

🍎 Was your morning coffee too hot for comfort? Swallow 2 teaspoons of olive oil to coat and soothe your scalded throat.

## REMARKABLE RECIPES

## FOOT SOOTHER & SMOOTHER

Say goodbye to rough, cracked skin on your feet with this soothing, smoothing solution.

**1 tbsp. of olive oil**
**1 tbsp. of almond oil**
**1 tsp. of wheat germ**

Combine the ingredients, and store in a bottle with a tight cap. Shake well before using. Rub generously into feet and heels, especially the dry areas. Your tootsies will love you for it!

# OLIVE OIL

## Home Cleaning & Upkeep

◆ Remove "rainbow" streaks from stainless steel by rubbing them with olive oil.

◆ Got salt stains on your silver saltshakers or other silver pieces? To clean them off, rub olive oil on the spots, let them sit for a few days, and wipe with a soft cotton cloth.

◆ Polish lacquered metal by wiping it with a few drops of olive oil.

◆ Do you have a string of pearls that's looking dingy? Put a dab of olive oil on a soft cloth, smooth it onto each pearl, and wipe with a second clean cloth.

◆ Use olive oil to make your patent leather bags and shoes shine. Clean the leather with a damp cloth, apply a few drops of olive oil on a clean cloth, and buff to a shine.

◆ Here's a recipe for wood floor polish that can't be beat: Mix equal amounts of olive oil and white vinegar in a spray bottle. Apply a thin mist to the floor, and rub it in well, using cotton rags or a wax applicator. Remove the excess polish with clean cotton rags, and buff to a shine. Be careful—the floor will be slippery at first.

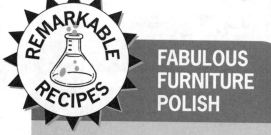

### REMARKABLE RECIPES

### FABULOUS FURNITURE POLISH

The next time you run out of furniture polish, don't buy more—use this simple, all-natural alternative instead.

**2 tbsp. of lemon juice**
**10 drops of lemon oil**
**4 drops of olive oil**

Mix the juice and the oils in a bowl, dip a soft cotton cloth into the mixture, and apply it gently to your furniture with a circular motion. The potion will nourish the wood and make it smell good, too!

# ONINONS

 Health & Beauty

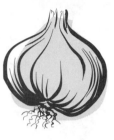

Have you (or your favorite teenager) broken out in pimples? Reach for this heirloom helper: Mix 1 teaspoon of onion juice with 2 tablespoons of honey, and apply it to your face. Wait 10 to 15 minutes, and rinse with warm water followed by cool water.

Ease the pain of a minor burn with an onion. First, run cold water over the burned area. Then apply a slice of raw onion. The same chemicals that make you cry also block the substances that make you feel pain. And here's a bonus: Onion juice has antibacterial properties that may help to prevent infection.

When you feel faint, hold a cut onion under your nose until the wooziness passes.

Relieve the itch and burn of athlete's foot by massaging onion juice into your tootsies twice a day.

Eliminate warts by rubbing them with half an onion that's been dipped in salt. Use this treatment twice a day until the warts disappear.

## TRASH TO TREASURE

HERE ARE some ways to put mesh onion bags to work:

○ Use a mesh bag and soapy water to scrub dead bugs off your windshield.

○ Tuck a bar of soap into a mesh bag, hang it on an outside faucet, and wash grimy hands with it—no need to remove the soap.

○ Wad up a mesh bag, put it in the bottom of a vase, and stick flower stems through the holes. They'll stay exactly where you want them.

## Home Cleaning & Upkeep

◆ To get rid of scuff marks on a tile floor, rub the spots with a pantyhose pouch filled with grated onion.

◆ Use the skins of yellow onions to dye eggs a pretty shade of orange. (See the recipe for simple dyes on page 262.)

◆ Has your favorite knife gotten rusty? Here's a great tip: Use it to slice up an onion or two, and it'll be as clean as a whistle.

◆ About to start a painting project? Eliminate eau de paint by dropping big chunks of raw onion in a pan of cold water and setting it in the middle of the room.

## REMARKABLE RECIPES

### GARLIC AND ONION JUICE

This aromatic elixir helps control pests on fruit, flower, and vegetable plants.

**2 cloves of garlic**
**2 medium onions**
**3 cups of water**

Put all of the ingredients in a blender, and whirl them up. Strain out the solids, pour the remaining liquid into a hand-held spray bottle, and use it whenever you need potent relief from soft-bodied insects. Bury the leftover solids in your garden to repel aphids and other pesky pests.

## Yard & Garden

● For easy mole control, tuck a wedge of onion into each run.

● To keep whiteflies from bugging your houseplants, use this simple mix: Grate the skin of 1 medium onion, put it in 2 cups of water, and let it steep overnight. Add 1 quart of warm water, and use it to spray your plants once a month.

# ORANGES & ORANGE JUICE

## Health & Beauty

Tame those flyaway hairs with this sweet spray. Finely chop one peeled orange. Add it to 2 cups of boiling water, and boil until about half of the original liquid remains. Cool, strain out the orange, and mix in 1 ounce of rubbing alcohol. Then pour the solution into a spray bottle, and store it in the refrigerator. It'll keep for two to three weeks. (If it turns sticky, add a little more water.)

Feeling sluggish? Try this cool, invigorating, and nourishing masque: Mix 1 teaspoon of plain yogurt with the juice of ¼ of an orange (about 2 tablespoons). Smooth the mixture onto your face, wait 5 minutes, and rinse.

Here's the perfect relaxer: Wrap a few chamomile tea bags in gauze or a pantyhose leg. Next, cut an orange into thin slices. Suspend the tea pouch under your bathtub spigot, and let warm water flow over it as it fills the tub. Float the orange slices in the water, climb into the tub, and soak your troubles away.

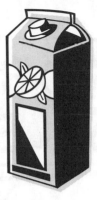

### REMARKABLE RECIPES

## OLD-TIME TUMMY TAMER

When nausea strikes, reach for this classic remedy.

**½ cup of fresh-squeezed orange juice**
**2 tbsp. of clear corn syrup**
**Pinch of salt**
**½ cup of water**

Mix all of the ingredients together, and store the potion in a covered jar in the refrigerator. Take 1 tablespoon every half-hour or so until your queasiness has flown the coop.

# Home Cleaning & Upkeep

◆ Getting ready to sell your house? Shortly before potential buyers are due to arrive, grab an orange and shave the peel. Then toss the shavings into a pot of boiling water, along with a handful of cloves and a few cinnamon sticks. Real estate surveys show that this spicy-sweet aroma is one of the two most likely to make house-hunters think, "This is the place!" (The other is fresh-baked bread.)

◆ Time to dye Easter eggs? Use orange peels to get a delicate, light yellow color. (See the easy directions on page 262.)

# Yard & Garden

● To send unwanted ants packing, purée equal parts of orange peels and water in a blender, and pour the mixture directly onto the colony early in the morning.

● Here's a simple, but lethal spray to use on caterpillars, aphids, whiteflies, and other soft-bodied pests: Put 1 cup of chopped orange peels in a blender, pour ¼ cup of boiling water over them, and liquefy. Let the mixture sit overnight at room temperature, and strain it through cheesecloth. Pour the liquid into a hand-held spray bottle, fill the balance of the bottle with water, and spray your plants from top to bottom.

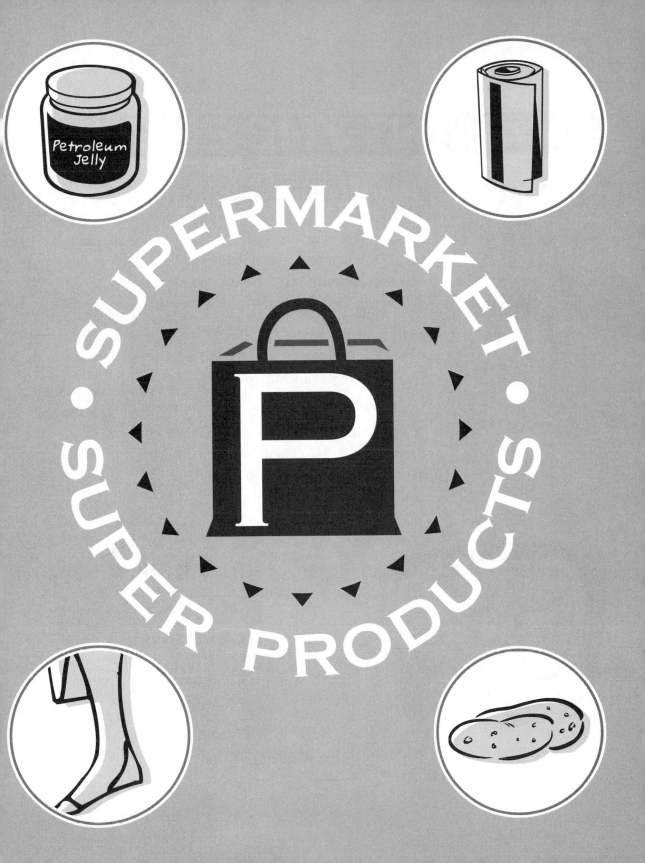

# P

# PANTYHOSE

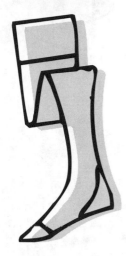

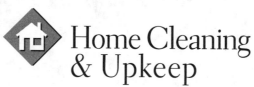 Health & Beauty

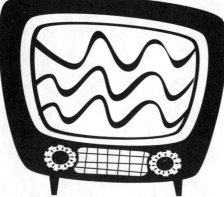 Instead of spending money on cotton or tissue, use pantyhose to remove nail polish. Just cut the old hose into 1-inch rings, and dampen them with polish remover.

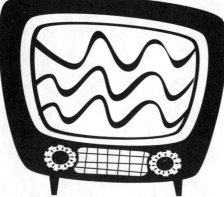 Put homemade cleansing grains and bath-time "teas" in pantyhose pouches. Use the cleansing-grain pouch for scrubbing all over. Soak the tea pouch in your tub to scent the water while you bathe.

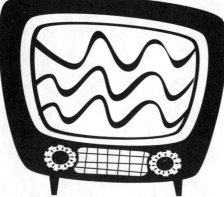 Make a back scrubber by cutting off a pantyhose leg, putting a bar of soap inside, and tying a knot at each side of the soap. Then, just hold one end of the hose in each hand, and scrub-a-dub-dub!

## Home Cleaning & Upkeep

◆ Clean metal mini-blinds, computer and television screens, and other dust "magnets" with pantyhose—which also attracts dust like nobody's business.

◆ Turn pantyhose into bags for holding odor- and dampness-chasing products like chalk and charcoal.

◆ Time to take down the Christmas tree? Before you start cleaning up the aftermath, use this trick to save yourself the hassle of a clogged vacuum cleaner: Put a pantyhose leg over the nozzle. The needles will stick to the nylon surface, instead of the inside of the vacuum. When you're through with the job, just peel off the stocking over a wastebasket, and throw the stocking and needles away.

◆ To vacuum dust from drawers, counters, or bookshelves without removing the contents, cover your vacuum cleaner nozzle with a piece of old pantyhose.

◆ Pull a pantyhose leg over your mop and use it to polish your floor.

◆ Use pantyhose as gentle scrubbers for windows, walls, furniture, and even non-stick cookware.

◆ Store onions or garlic in a pantyhose leg. Drop in a bulb, tie a knot, drop another one in, and so on. When you want to use one of the bulbs, cut just below the knot above it.

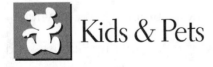

## Kids & Pets

■ Make a can't-leave-it-alone cat toy with pantyhose. Just stuff a toe with catnip, and tie it shut.

■ Use pantyhose as sturdy, washable filler when you make stuffed animals for kids or dogs.

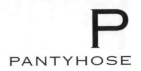
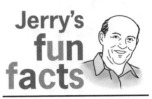

**Jerry's fun facts**

On May 15, 1940, nylon stockings first hit store shelves all over the U.S.A. Women lined up for hours before the stores opened, and then stormed in like the 7th Cavalry. By the end of the year, consumers had bought 36 million pairs of nylon stockings. They'd have bought more, but there were none left. Pantyhose entered the picture almost two decades later, in 1958.

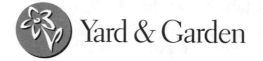 Yard & Garden

● Protect peach and nectarine trees from peach-leaf curl by hanging pantyhose pouches filled with moth balls from the limbs.

● Keep gladiolus and other tender bulbs dry and healthy through the winter. Just dust them with medicated baby powder, drop them into a pantyhose leg, and hang it in a cool, dry place.

● Make compost tea or manure tea by filling a pantyhose leg with the material and steeping it in 5 to 10 gallons of water for several days.

● Tie up vines and floppy plants with strips of pantyhose. As a bonus, the nylon will attract static electricity, which will give your plants added grow power.

● Deter nasty vine borers by wrapping pantyhose around the base of each melon, squash, and cucumber plant. The moths generally lay their eggs in these lower reaches, and if they find the stem covered, they'll probably go elsewhere.

● Anytime you mix up disease- and pest-control potions, strain them through a piece of pantyhose to catch any solid ingredients.

● Cover ripening fruits and vegetables in your garden with pantyhose to protect them from nibbling rodents, birds, and insects.

# PAPER PRODUCTS

## 🏠 Home Cleaning & Upkeep

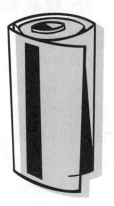

◆ To clean hardened mineral deposits from around faucets, cover them with paper towels that are saturated with vinegar. Leave the towels in place for about 2 hours. The deposits will wipe right off.

◆ Candle wax melted on your table top? Put a ⅛-inch-thick layer of paper towels on top of the wax, then apply an iron set on warm/hot. The wax should be absorbed into the paper. If any remains on the table, scrape it off with a piece of cardboard or a plastic knife.

◆ Do you dread the thought of cleaning a broiler pan? Don't! The next time you broil meat, before you sit down to dinner, lay a paper towel in the dirty pan. Squirt dishwashing liquid on the towel, then saturate it with hot water. Let it soak while you dine. When you've finished eating, all you'll have to do is wipe the pan clean.

◆ After oiling your sewing machine, prevent nasty oil stains by stitching several rows on a sheet of paper towel before you work on fabric.

◆ When you stack cast-iron skillets in a cupboard, separate them with paper towels to absorb moisture and prevent rust from forming in the skillets.

◆ Out of coffee filters? Roll a double layer of paper towels into a cone, and use that instead.

# P
## PAPER PRODUCTS

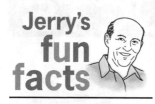

◆ To keep vegetables fresher longer, line your refrigerator's produce bin with paper towels to absorb excess moisture.

◆ Do you have a book that got caught in the rain? Here's how to prevent wrinkles and mildew: Slide paper towels between the damp pages, close the book, and set a heavier book on top. Let it sit overnight. If it's still not dry, repeat the process, replacing the towels with fresh ones.

◆ Use paper towels to remove candle wax from carpet or upholstery. Lay a thick layer of towels over the wax, and gently press with a warm iron. The iron will melt the wax, and the paper towel will absorb it.

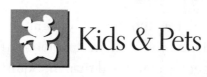 ## Kids & Pets

■ Here's a simple way to put patterned, one-of-a-kind eggs into the kids' Easter baskets. First, lay a paper towel over a piece of aluminum foil. Then dribble 8 to 10 drops of food coloring on the towel. (For a more intricate design, repeat with more colors.) Set a damp, hard-cooked egg on top, and gently wrap the paper and foil around the egg. Wait a few seconds, then open the "package" and let the egg dry.

■ Need to decorate a birthday cake, but there's no time to frost it? Put a clean paper doily on top of the cake, and dust it with some confectioners' sugar or unsweetened cocoa powder. Gently lift off the doily, and voilà—a masterpiece!

# Yard & Garden

● Use wax-paper cups to keep rain from destroying the smell of deer deterrents such as soap, hair, or ammonia-scented rags. Here's how: Put the material into an old pantyhose foot, and tie it closed with a string. Poke a hole in the bottom of a 12-ounce drink cup, tuck the pouch inside, pull the string through the hole, and fasten it to a tree branch. The aroma should stay fresh for about a year.

● Keep marauding raccoons and other critters out of your garbage cans by dipping a large wad of paper towels in ammonia, dowsing with hot sauce, and tossing the paper into the can.

● Control cutworms by making plant collars out of paper cups. Punch out the bottoms, and push the cups about 2 inches into the ground, leaving 3 inches showing above.

● To make your own seed-starting tape, use toilet paper. Just stretch out a length that's convenient to work with, dampen your seeds, and space them at the proper planting distance. Put another layer of toilet paper on top. Carefully roll up the paper to carry it to your prepared bed. Set it in the bed, cover it with soil to the depth that's right for your seeds, and water.

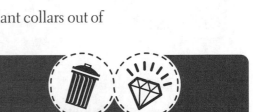

## TRASH TO TREASURE

HERE'S A useful tip for all of you who pick up youngsters after school or daycare: Keep a few empty paper towel rolls in the car. They're just the ticket for transporting works of art or scrapbook-quality exams to your home safely.

# P

# PETROLEUM JELLY

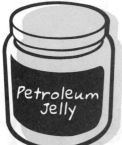

Petroleum Jelly

## Health & Beauty

Use petroleum jelly as a hair moisturizer and setting lotion. Rub a small amount between your palms, smooth it over your hair, and style it any way you like.

Are dry, chapped lips driving you crazy? Do what doctors recommend: Reach for petroleum jelly. The medical pros say it beats any commercial lip balm, hands down! If you find the greasiness uncomfortable for all-day use, smear on petroleum jelly before you go to bed at night, and use lip balm during your waking hours.

Here's how to make your own tinted, flavored lip gloss. In a bowl, mix 1 tablespoon of petroleum jelly, ¼ teaspoon of lipstick, and two to four drops of your favorite extract—for instance, orange, rum, or peppermint. Then scrape the gloss into a small, lidded container (an empty 35-mm film canister is perfect).

If you discover that a lipstick you've recently bought is too dark, add a little petroleum jelly to subdue the color and add instant shine.

## REMARKABLE RECIPES

### ACHING MUSCLE MAGIC

Ease your sore, aching muscles with this minty remedy.

**1 tbsp. of petroleum jelly**
**6 drops of peppermint oil**
**Warm water**

Mix the oil and jelly in a small bowl; put it in a larger bowl of warm water. Soak a towel in warm tap water, wring it out, and drape it over the trouble spot. After 3 minutes, remove the towel, and rub the oil/jelly mixture into your skin.

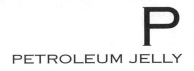

Your eyeliner will flow on more smoothly if you dip it in petroleum jelly first.

Get pierced earrings in your ears more gently by coating the posts with a little petroleum jelly before you insert them.

Prevent hangnails by rubbing petroleum jelly into your (or your child's) cuticles.

Tired of struggling to open nail polish bottles? Smear a little petroleum jelly on the inside of the cap and the rim of the bottle before you've used it. The cap will come right off every time. (This trick works with tubes of glue, too.)

To make the scent of your perfume last longer, simply spread a very thin layer of petroleum jelly on your skin before you dab on the fragrance.

You can moisturize and soften your eyelashes by giving them a thin coat of petro-leum jelly at bedtime each night.

To make a razor blade last up to 5 times longer, dry it well after each use, coat it with a thin layer of petroleum jelly, and wipe off any excess—*very* carefully, please!

Rub petroleum jelly on your cheeks before going out in the cold, to prevent chapping.

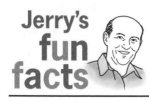

In 1859, a Brooklyn chemist named Robert Chesebrough acquired a few jars of petroleum residue that kept clogging up the drilling rods at a Pennsylvania oil field. He was able to extract and purify the gunk's essential ingredient—a substance he called "petroleum jelly." By 1870, he was manufacturing Vaseline®. Mr. Chesebrough lived to be 96, and said he owed his longevity to the fact that he ate a spoonful of Vaseline® every day!

# 🏠 Home Cleaning & Upkeep

◆ Keep patent leather shoes, bags, and belts smooth and shiny by rubbing them with petroleum jelly.

◆ To remove white water spots from leather, cover them with a thick coat of petroleum jelly. Leave it on for a day or so, and wipe it off with a soft cloth.

◆ How's this for an easy fire starter? Just dip a few cotton balls in petroleum jelly, and set them into your barbecue grill or campfire. One match will set them ablaze, and they'll burn hot enough to get even the dampest kindling going strong.

◆ Got a squeaky door hinge that's driving you nuts? Take a fingertipful of petroleum jelly, rub it into the hinge, and open and close the door a few times to work the jelly in. Wipe off the excess with a cloth, and that squeak will squawk no more!

◆ Tired of struggling to get melted wax out of candlesticks? Coat the insides of the holders with petroleum jelly *before* you insert the candles. The wax will slide right out.

◆ Quiet a screeching faucet with petroleum jelly. Just remove the handle and stem, coat the metal threads, and screw the pieces back together.

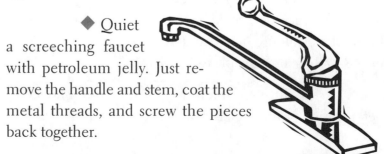

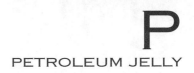

◆ Use petroleum jelly to remove stains, minor scratches, and water rings from wooden furniture. Simply smear on a thick coat, let it sit for 24 hours, and rub it in thoroughly. Wipe away the excess, and polish as usual.

◆ Does moisture make your outdoor light-bulbs stick when you try to remove them? Before you insert a new bulb, rub a light coat of petroleum jelly in and on the threads.

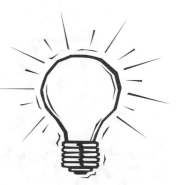

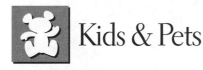 ## Kids & Pets

■ Has dry winter air left your dog's feet cracked and sore? Soothe and soften those paws by massaging a little petroleum jelly into the pads and between the toes.

■ You want to pass your old fielder's mitt on to your child or grandchild, but the leather has dried out? Rub petroleum jelly into it. That glove will be as soft and supple as ever!

■ Petroleum jelly can help you break in a new glove, too. Massage the jelly into the leather, put a baseball in the palm, and tie the glove closed around it. Leave it for a day or two, untie the cord, and presto—a mitt that's ready for your little slugger's first triple play!

■ Keep shampoo out of baby's (or Fido's) eyes by rubbing a thin line of petroleum jelly above the eyebrows. The suds will roll off to the side, which means no more tears!

■ To remove gum from a child's (or a pet's) hair, apply a thick coat of petroleum jelly, and work it in with your fingers until the gum slides out.

■ Are the kids giving a show that has a *very* sad scene in it? Have them dab petroleum jelly down their cheeks to simulate tears.

■ Lubricate the wheels of roller skates and skateboards by smearing petroleum jelly around the cylinders. They'll roll a lot faster!

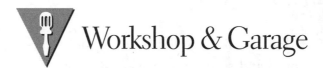

## Workshop & Garage

▼ For a super shine, rub petroleum jelly onto your car's leather or vinyl interior.

▼ Smear petroleum jelly onto car battery terminals to prevent corrosion. (Be sure to clean them first!)

▼ Keep outdoor machinery from rusting by coating all metal parts with petroleum jelly.

▼ This routine is sure to make after-painting cleanup a breeze: Before you start the job, dip a cotton swab in petroleum jelly, and rub it along the edges of windows, doorknobs, hinges, and other hardware. And spread a thin coat of the jelly along tile or linoleum floors. Then for good measure, rub your hands all over with petroleum jelly. When you call it quits for the day, any paint smears and splatters will slide right off!

# POTATOES

 ## Health & Beauty

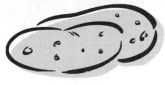

Potato juice reduces inflammation caused by eczema. Just grate a raw potato, dip a cotton pad in the shreds to absorb some of the juice, and gently dab the trouble spots.

To reduce bags and dark circles under your eyes, grate a raw potato, and wrap the shavings in two pieces of cheesecloth or two pantyhose pouches. Lie down, put one sack over each eye, and relax for 15 minutes. Repeat daily, until the circles fade. (If you don't mind the messiness, you can dispense with the cloth and apply the potatoes directly to your skin as a poultice.)

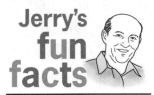

Been out berry-picking? Get the stains off of your hands by rubbing the skin with a slice of raw potato and rinsing with clear water.

Give your hair brunette highlights with this routine: Cook an unpeeled potato in boiling water until the water has colored. Turn off the heat, leave the potato in the pot, and let the water cool until it is tepid. Dip a pastry brush into the water, and use it to saturate your hair (being careful not to get any water in your eyes or on your skin). Leave the potato water on your hair for 30 minutes, and rinse thoroughly with cool water. Repeat every few weeks to retain the highlights.

Although tomatoes top the list of most-grown vegetables in American gardens, the most-eaten award goes to potatoes. Statistics show that we consume two spuds for every tomato. Or, to put it in more graphic terms, the average American gobbles up a whopping 126 pounds of taters each year!

# P

## POTATOES

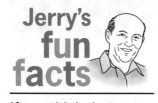
 Coax a splinter out of your skin with a raw potato. Tape a slice onto the affected site, or if the sliver is in your finger or toe, hollow out a space that's just the right size, and slip the digit into the spud. (Hold it in place with a sock if you need to.) Leave the tater in place overnight, and you'll be able to easily pluck the splinter out in the morning.

 Soothe a minor burn by rubbing it gently with the cut surface of a raw potato.

## Home Cleaning & Upkeep

◆ Got some mud on your cotton or synthetic clothing? Rub the spots with a slice of raw potato, and toss the clothes into the wash. The dirt will come right out.

◆ Here's an old-time way to remove a broken lightbulb that's still in the socket. *First, make sure the power to the fixture is turned off!* Next, push half of a potato, cut side first, against the broken bulb. Turn the tater just as you would to unscrew a whole lightbulb. Once it's out of the socket, don't try to remove the bulb from the potato — just throw it all in the trash!

◆ If your scuffed shoes just won't take a shine, rub them with a raw potato, and then polish them as usual.

◆ To deodorize your refrigerator, cut a raw potato in two, and set both halves inside, cut side up. When the tater surfaces turn black, just shave off the discolored layer, and put the clean sections back on the job.

# Yard & Garden

● Before you plant a tree, line the hole with baking potatoes. They'll hold moisture that the young plant needs to get a healthy start. Later, as the taters decay, they'll provide essential nutrients to the growing tree.

● To get rid of mice, set out shallow containers of instant mashed potatoes, with a dish of water nearby. The mice will eat the potato powder, drink the water, swell up, and die.

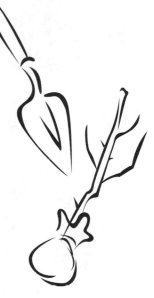

● Are slugs crawling up the sides of your flowerpots? Trap the pests by putting slices of raw potato around the bottom of each container. During the night, the slugs will zero in on the taters. In the morning, pick them up and drop them in a bag of salt.

● Trap wireworms by spearing chunks of potato on sticks that are about 8 inches long and burying them so that about 3 inches of each stick shows above ground. Every week or so, pull up the chunks, toss them in a pail of soapy water to kill the worms, and empty the contents of the pail onto the compost pile.

● Use a raw potato to transport cuttings for short distances. Just cut a slice off an end of the potato, poke holes in it using a chopstick or thin twig, and insert your cuttings. They'll stay moist and fresh for several hours.

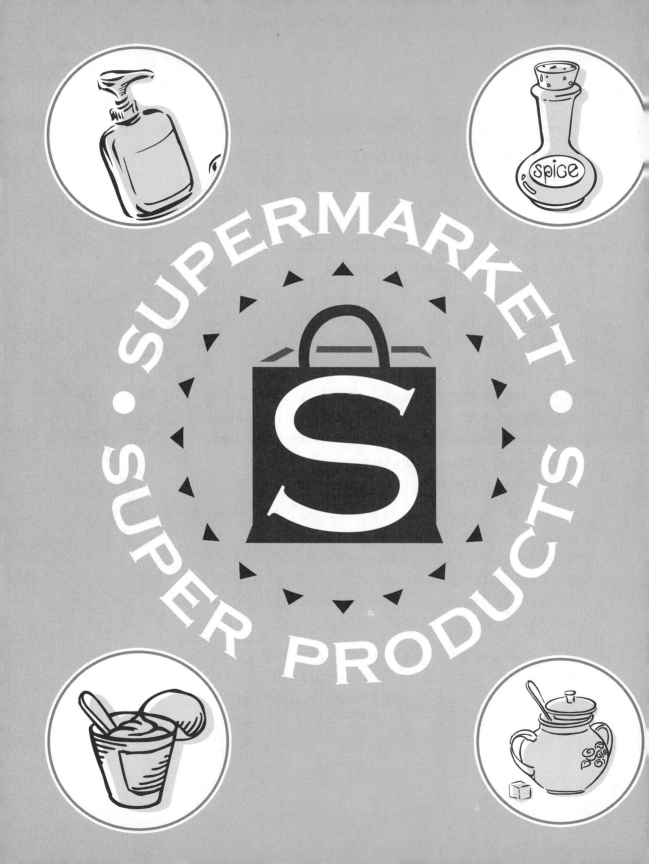

# SALT

 Health & Beauty

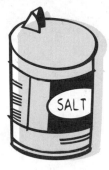

 When summer turns steamy, do you sweat buckets? Keep your cool by drinking plenty of water, and add ½ teaspoon of salt to every quart. And start downing the fluids *before* you feel thirsty, because your body needs water before your brain knows it.

 If your new dentures or braces are a little bit uncomfortable, toughen up your gums by gargling with a solution of 1 to 2 teaspoons of salt in a glass of warm water. (But if your mouth is still tender after a few days of this treatment, call your orthodontist or dentist.)

 Need fast relief from sunburn? Mix 1 to 2 teaspoons of salt in a glass of ice-cold milk, and sponge the solution onto your skin once or twice a day until the pain is gone.

 Looking for a masque that will tighten up enlarged pores? This one couldn't be simpler: Mix a little buttermilk and table salt into a paste. Apply it to your face, and massage well. Leave it on for about 5 minutes, rinse with warm water, and pat dry.

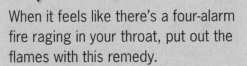

## SORE THROAT GARGLE

When it feels like there's a four-alarm fire raging in your throat, put out the flames with this remedy.

**1 clove of garlic**
**1 tsp. of salt**
**1 tiny pinch of cayenne pepper**
**1 large glass of water**

Crush the garlic clove and put it into the glass. Add the salt, pepper, and water, and stir. Then gargle with the solution. Repeat as needed, but if your throat doesn't feel better in a day or so, call your doctor.

 Before summer sandal time rolls around, start softening up your feet with a simple salt rub. Just add a few drops of your favorite scented oil to 2 tablespoons or so of warm water, and mix in enough salt to make a paste. Pat the mixture onto your feet, rub with a washcloth for 2 to 3 minutes, and rinse.

 Are your feet just plain tired? Soak those dogs in a basin of salty water. Use about 1 cup of salt per gallon of warm water.

 Out of toothpaste? Use salt instead. Just pour a little into the palm of your hand, dip a moist toothbrush into it, and brush away.

## Home Cleaning & Upkeep

 Before you use a new broom for the first time, soak the bristles in hot salt water. The broom will sweep cleaner, longer. (This works only on natural-bristle brooms, though—not plastic.)

 To remove cat urine from a carpet, pour a thick layer of salt on the wet spot. Make sure you use plenty—the salt will only pull out as much liquid as it can hold. Let it sit overnight, or until the salt has hardened. Sweep up as much as you can, then vacuum up the rest. (If a stain remains, it means you didn't use enough salt.)

◆ Use salt to clean your oven. Treat fresh spills this way: After you've turned the oven off, but while it's still hot, cover the stain completely with salt. Wait until the oven has cooled completely, and go at the spill with a rubber spatula or non-scratch scouring pad. That old food will crumble away.

◆ If an oven spill has already cooled and hardened *before* you've had a chance to tackle it, dampen the stain with water, sprinkle salt on top, and scrub with a non-scratch scouring pad.

◆ Are your copper-bottomed pots and pans stained and splotchy? Try this wonder-working routine: Mix a few teaspoons of salt with enough vinegar to make a gritty paste. Apply it with your fingers or a sponge, and work it in with a fine (00) steel-wool pad. Rinse with clear water. Repeat every month or so to keep your pots and pans gleaming.

◆ Has starch built up on your iron? To get it off, just put a paper towel on the ironing board, sprinkle salt on top of it, and move the hot iron over the salt in a circular motion for a minute or so. This will gently scrub the bottom clean. When the iron has cooled down, wipe away any residue with a damp cloth.

◆ Use salt to clean bottles that have hard-to-reach "shoulders." Just pour ½ teaspoon or so of salt into the bottle, and plug the top with a cork or a wad of paper towel. Shake, rattle, and roll the bottle until it's spotless, and rinse with clear water.

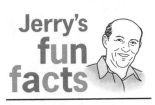

**Jerry's fun facts**

When payday rolls around, do you think about salt? Probably not. But early Roman soldiers did, because part of their earnings came in the form of special salt rations. They were known as *salarium argentum,* and that's where we got our English word *salary.* So, come next payday, maybe you *will* think of salt!

◆ Are you what a friend of mine calls a WWFF (White Wicker Furniture Fiend)? If so, this tip's just for you: To keep your treasures as white as snow without painting, mix ¼ cup of salt in 1 gallon of warm water. Dip a stiff brush into the solution, give the furniture a good scrubbing, and let it dry in the sun.

◆ To remove rust from knives, cast-iron pans, or other kitchen gear, make a paste from 2 parts salt and 1 part lemon juice. Rub the paste onto the metal until the spots vanish, and rinse with clear water.

◆ When damp laundry sits too long in hot weather and winds up with mold or mildew, act fast—*before* the spots become permanent stains. Mix up a paste of roughly equal parts of lemon juice and salt, rub it into the splotches, and wash the load again with your regular detergent.

◆ This trick will make your pantyhose and stockings wear better and last longer: Before you put them on for the first time, soak them for 1 to 3 hours in a solution made of ½ cup of salt per quart of water. Then wash them in mild, soapy water, and hang them up to dry.

◆ If you like your blue jeans to stay a dark, rich blue but lose that stiff-as-a-board texture, here's a tip for you: When you wash a pair of jeans for the first time, add ¼ cup of salt to the wash cycle. It will help lock in the color *and* soften the fabric.

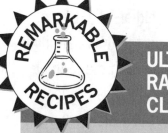

**REMARKABLE RECIPES**

## ULTIMATE RANGE CLEANER

When your stove top is covered in spaghetti sauce splatters and who-knows-what-else, reach for this range remedy.

**3 tbsp. of salt**
**3 tbsp. of baking soda**
**Pinch of cream of tartar**
**Hydrogen peroxide**

Combine the salt, baking soda, and cream of tartar in a bowl. Add enough hydrogen peroxide to make a paste. Spread the paste on the stains and let it sit for a half-hour or so, then scrub with a sponge dipped in warm water. Wipe off with a clean sponge.

◆ Remove perspiration stains from cotton clothes by soaking them in a solution of 1 to 2 cups of salt per gallon of water. Leave the duds in the brine for an hour or so, wring them out, and launder as usual.

◆ Despite their name, clothes moth larvae don't just attack clothing. They go after any fiber that has stains in it—sweat, urine, food, oil, starch—whatever. And that includes fibers in carpets and area rugs. So how do you get rid of the rascals? Simple: Sprinkle your carpets with a healthy layer of salt, then vacuum it up. Salt destroys moth larvae.

◆ Spilled some red wine on your best tablecloth? Don't worry. Just moisten the spot with water, sprinkle salt over it, let it sit for a few minutes (or until after dinner), and wash the tablecloth as usual.

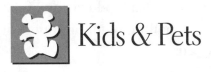

## Kids & Pets

■ When it's time to clean the fish tank, say a loud "No!" to soap—any residue it leaves behind could kill your fish. The same goes for other household cleansers. So how do you make that glass sparkle? Reach for the salt, a sponge, and hot water. Clean as you would with any scouring powder, and rinse thoroughly with clear, cool water.

■ Is it flea season again? Kill the tiny terrors by pouring salt into all the cracks in wood floors and baseboards.

■ To make a carpet flea-free, salt it at a rate of 6 pounds of salt per 100 square feet of rug. Wait 24 hours, and scrub with strong soap or carpet cleaner.

■ Give area rugs and your dog's bed cover the anti-flea treatment by washing them as usual, and then adding ½ cup of salt to the final rinse water.

## Yard & Garden

● To rout stubborn weeds from between the stones in your driveway or patio, upend a salt shaker and sprinkle away. Just be sure to aim *away* from any plants you want to leave standing, or they'll shrivel up along with the weeds! If you live in gusty territory, or you're not too sure about your aim, use this weed-killing method instead: Add ¼ cup of salt to 1 gallon of boiling water, and pour it over the weeds.

● When you're being visited by an army of ants, indoors or out, sprinkle salt on their trails. They'll scurry in a hurry!

● Are your hands grimy with garden soil? Add about a teaspoon of salt to the soap lather as you wash up, and they'll come out as clean as a whistle.

### REMARKABLE RECIPES

### LUXURIOUS BATH OIL

After a long, hard day in the yard (or even a short, easy one), nothing feels better than sinking into a tub full of hot water and this toddy for the body.

**2 cups of milk**
**1 cup of salt**
**1 cup of honey**
**¼ cup of baking soda**
**½ cup of baby oil**

Combine the milk, salt, honey, and baking soda in a large bowl. Fill your bathtub with water, pour in the mixture, and then add the baby oil (and, if you'd like, a few drops of your own favorite fragrance).

# SHAMPOO

 ## Home Cleaning & Upkeep

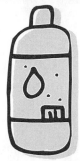

◆ Running low on laundry soap? Use plain ol' shampoo instead. It works especially well for delicate clothes. Less than half a cup will usually do a full load.

◆ Are you fresh out of dishwashing liquid? Reach for the shampoo (non-conditioning), and wash the dishes with that. It will cut right through grease and oil.

◆ Do you have ring-around-the-collar? Rub a little plain shampoo into the fabric, and the stains will all come out in the wash.

◆ Whoops! You (or a well-meaning helper) accidentally sent your best wool sweater through the washing machine, and now it's a shapeless lump. Is it ruined? Maybe. But before you give up hope, soak the sweater in tepid water with a squirt or two of good-quality shampoo added to it. This may soften the fibers enough to let you re-shape the garment. Stretch it out and shape it as best you can, then lay it flat to dry.

**REMARKABLE RECIPES**

## BRING ON THE BUBBLES!

If your idea of relaxation is sinking into a tub full of bubbles, then this recipe's for you!

**1 gal. of water**
**2 cups of soap flakes**
**½ cup of glycerin**
**2 cups of shampoo**
**Scented oil (optional)**

Mix the water, soap, and 2 table-spoons of the glycerin in a pot over low heat, stirring until the soap flakes have dissolved. In a large bowl, add this mixture to the rest of the glycerin, the shampoo and, if you'd like, scented oil. Store in quart containers at room temperature. To use, add 1 cup to the water as your tub is filling.

◆ Don't buy special, expensive detergents to clean your hand-washable silks and woolen knits—use shampoo instead. Just a drop or two mixed in cool water will do the trick.

◆ Wash hairbrushes and combs in a capful of shampoo in a sink filled with warm water. Let them soak for a few minutes, swish them around in the water, and rinse with clear water.

# Yard & Garden

● To keep pesky birds from getting to your fruit before you do, spray your fruit-filled bushes and trees with a solution of 1 tablespoon of baby shampoo and 1 tablespoon of ammonia in 1 gallon of water. Repeat after each rain. Make sure to rinse the fruit thoroughly when you're ready to eat it.

● Getting ready to sow seed for a new lawn? Before you start, put the grass seeds in a container with a mixture of ¼ cup of baby shampoo, 1 tablespoon of Epsom salts, and 1 gallon of weak tea. Put the container in the refrigerator for two days, then sift out the seeds, let them dry, and sow as usual. You'll see almost 100 percent germination—*guaranteed!*

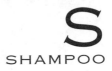

● Stop powdery mildew before it starts by spraying your trouble-prone plants once a week with a mix of 2 tablespoons of baby shampoo and 1 tablespoon of baking soda in 1 gallon of warm water.

● Maintain the vivid color of your houseplants by mist-spraying the foliage every week or so with a mixture of 1 twice-used tea bag, 1 teaspoon of antiseptic mouthwash, 3 teaspoons of mild shampoo, and 3 teaspoons of ammonia in a quart of warm water.

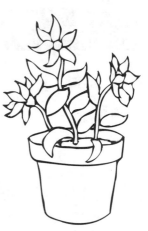

● When winter is heading in fast, and your garden is still full of un-ripe veggies, get the show on the road with this routine: Mix 1 cup of apple juice, ½ cup of baby shampoo, and ½ cup of ammonia in your 20 gallon hose-end sprayer jar. Fill the balance of the jar with warm water, and spray your plants to the point of run-off.

● Get garden-variety grime off of your hands by washing them with shampoo. It's especially effective at re-moving grease and oil that you've picked up from the lawn mower or from freshly lubricated tools.

● Keep whiteflies under con-trol by spraying garden plants with a mix of 2 tablespoons of baby shampoo in 1 gallon of water. Spray your plants liber-ally, paying attention to the undersides of leaves, where the little buggers hide out.

## REMARKABLE RECIPES

### BULB BATH

To keep your bulbs healthy and bug-free, treat them to this nice, warm bath before tucking them into their planting bed.

**2 tsp. of baby shampoo**
**1 tsp. of antiseptic mouthwash**
**¼ tsp. of instant tea granules**
**2 gal. of warm water**

Mix all of the ingredients in a bucket, and carefully set your bulbs into the solution. Stir gently, then remove the bulbs one at a time, and plant them. When you're through, serve the nutri-tious bathwater to a thirsty tree or parched shrub.

# SOAP

## Health & Beauty

Fresh out of ingredients for a fancy facial cleansing masque? Use this simple recipe instead: Mix liquid hand soap with enough salt to make a paste. Dab it onto your face (don't rub!), wait 2 minutes, and rinse with clear water.

If you have dry skin, use this pampering treatment: Pour a little liquid castile soap into the palm of your hand, and add about 1 teaspoon of honey. Massage it into your face until it lathers, being careful to avoid your eyes. Rinse with warm water, and pat dry.

It's easy to make your own shampoo. Mix ¼ cup of liquid castile soap and ½ teaspoon of light vegetable oil in ¼ cup of water. Pour the mixture into a clean, empty pump or squeeze bottle, and you're ready to roll. (If your hair is very oily, omit the vegetable oil.)

Got a mosquito or spider bite? Rub a wet bar of soap directly on the spot. The itch will vanish quickly, and the swelling will soon disappear, too.

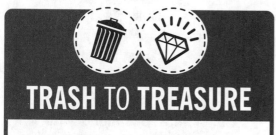

## TRASH TO TREASURE

**DON'T THROW** away those soap wrappers, folks! Instead, tuck them into dresser drawers and linen cupboards to keep the contents smelling clean and fresh.

If you or your family members work out at a gym, you know how stinky those gym bags can get—so keep 'em fresh by tossing in a soap wrapper.

When you need to draw a bee's stinger out of your skin, rub a bar of soap over the area. The buzzer's weapon should slide right out.

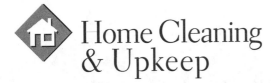

# Home Cleaning & Upkeep

What do you do when you get all set up to sew something and discover that you're fresh out of dressmaker's chalk? Use white bar soap to mark your fabric instead.

Wrap a scrap of cloth around a bar of soap, fasten it on the bottom with tape, and use it as a pincushion. The soap will lubricate the pins and needles, so they'll glide right through any kind of fabric. The cloth cover makes for a neater appearance, and also keeps the soap from sliding around.

Wrap a few new bars of soap loosely in facial tissue, and tuck them into drawers and linen cupboards to keep the contents smelling fresh.

Are your windows and drawers hard to open? Rub the gliders with a bar of soap to make them slide more easily.

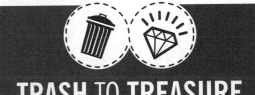

## TRASH TO TREASURE

THERE ARE lots of products made for getting out clothing stains, including those convenient stain sticks. But here's a little secret—stains rubbed with plain old soap come out clean just as often as those on clothes that got the stick treatment. So don't toss out those slivers and ends of bar soap. Just moisten the piece of soap with a drop of water, and dab any stains on clothes that are on their way to the laundry basket. You'll save a fortune on those specialty treatments!

◆ Do you love to cook over an open fire, but hate the chore of getting the soot off of the pans afterwards? Try this trick: Before you start cooking, rub a bar of soap over the bottom of each pan. When dinner's over, cleanup will be a breeze!

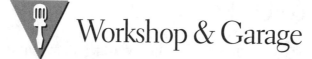

# Workshop & Garage

▼ Want to fog-proof your car's windows? It's a snap: Just rub a bar of soap over the glass, and polish it with a clean, soft cloth. This trick works just as well on diving masks and ski goggles, too.

▼ Are you doing some carpentry work with thin or brittle wood? Keep it from splitting by lubricating the nails with soap before you go ahead and pound them in.

▼ Before you cut wood with a handsaw, rub a bar of soap across the blade. It will make the job easier and the cut smoother.

▼ When you paint around windows, nix the need for any tape or scraping by running a bar of soap around the panes. Any splattered paint will wipe right up. Just be sure not to soap the wood!

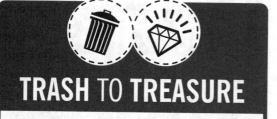

## TRASH TO TREASURE

**WHEN YOUR** bar of soap dwindles down to a sliver, don't throw it out! Instead, set it aside until you've got a handful of pieces, and stuff them into a pantyhose leg. Hang your soap sack from the outdoor water faucet, and use it to wash your hardworking hands. Or, dangle the bag under running water in the bathtub, and you'll have an instant bubble bath.

# SOUR CREAM & YOGURT

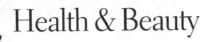 Health & Beauty

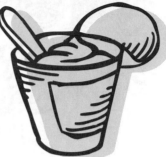

Is your skin normal to oily? If the answer is yes, then soften and nourish your face with this formula: Purée half a cucumber in a blender, and mix in 1 tablespoon of plain yogurt. Apply the mixture to your face, wait 30 minutes, and rinse with warm water.

When it comes to moisturizing dry skin, this masque can't be beet, er, beat. Just whirl 1 grated beet and 1 cup of sour cream in a blender, and smooth the mixture over your face and neck. Wait 10 minutes or so, and rinse with warm water.

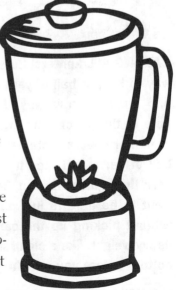

Need some scrubbing action? Try this nutritious facial cleanser: Grind about 1 tablespoon of dry oatmeal in the coffee grinder until it's a fine powder. If your skin is normal to oily, mix the oats with about 2 tablespoons of unflavored yogurt; for dry skin, use 2 tablespoons of sour cream. Wash your face with the mixture, and rinse with warm water.

Troubled by canker sores? Heal them the good-tasting way—by eating yogurt twice a day! Just make sure you choose a brand that has live *Lactobacillus acidophilus* cultures in it, because that's what kills the bacteria that cause the sores.

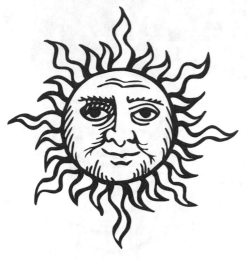

 For surefire sunburn relief, reach for cold, plain yogurt, and slather it on your skin. It works like a charm to lower the heat and take away the pain.

 Ladies, if you just can't keep yeast infections at bay, take a tip from the folks at the *Annals of Internal Medicine,* and eat more yogurt! The journal has reported that simply eating yogurt every day heightens resistance to *Candida albicans,* the bacteria that cause the infections. Again, though, look for those active cultures (*Lactobacillus acidophilus*) on the label.

 This easy conditioner will add protein and body to your hair: Beat the white of 1 egg until it's foamy, and stir it into 5 tablespoons of plain, natural yogurt. Apply the mixture to one small section of your hair at a time. Leave it in for 15 minutes, and rinse.

 Is the skin on your feet dry and rough? Treat yourself to this simple softening routine: First, soak your feet in warm water for 10 to 15 minutes, and dry them with a soft towel. Next, rub cornmeal into your feet, paying special attention to the driest parts, then rinse. Finally, massage your feet with a mixture of ½ cup of chilled sour cream and 2 tablespoons of olive oil. Rinse with warm water, and pat dry.

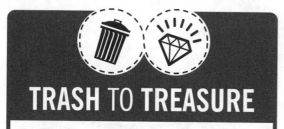

## TRASH TO TREASURE

**CALLING ALL knitters! Here's a terrific way to keep a ball of yarn tangle-free and out of harm's way. Just poke a hole in the lid of a well-washed sour cream or yogurt container, drop in the ball of yarn, and feed the end of the yarn through the hole in the lid. If you want to be able to just pull the yarn without picking up the carton, put a heavy weight, like a clean stone, in the bottom before you add the yarn.**

## Home Cleaning & Upkeep

◆ Are your piano keys looking almost as yellow as the rose of Texas? Tickle those ivories with a dab of plain yogurt on a soft cotton cloth. When you're through, they'll shine like the harvest moon!

◆ If you've scraped the price tags from the cases of your new CDs, but the glue won't budge, reach for sour cream or yogurt. Put a dab on a paper towel, and wipe the sticky spot. It'll vanish like magic.

## Kids & Pets

■ Oral antibiotics some-times cause stomachaches and diarrhea in pets, just as in humans. So, when the vet puts Fido or Fluffy (or Bunny) on meds, add yogurt to your pal's diet. You want a brand that contains live cultures, because they'll restore the beneficial bac-teria that antibiotics destroy in the process of killing the disease-causing organisms.

■ Give your dog a big nutri-tional boost without expensive supple-ments: Just add a little yogurt to his diet. A teaspoon a day, mixed with his regular kibble, will do the trick.

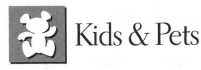

**REMARKABLE RECIPES**

### FROZEN BIRD TREATS

Want to give your pet bird a cool and healthy treat? Whip up a batch of these goodies.

**1 qt. (32 oz.) of vanilla yogurt**
**1 cup of mashed fruit***
**2 tbsp. of peanut butter**
**2 tbsp. of honey**

Mix all of the ingredients in a blender, and freeze the mixture in ice cube trays or 3-ounce paper cups. When Polly wants a snack, just nuke one treat for a few seconds, and serve.

*Or substitute 1 large jar of baby fruit.*

# S

## SPICES

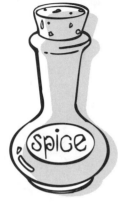

### ✚ Health & Beauty

🌿 To relieve a cough, pop a clove into your mouth, and suck on it. The tingly taste tends to ease throat tickles better than sweet cough drops or syrups. Sucking on a dried clove or two has another advantage—it'll make your breath smell spicy-sweet.

🌿 Attempting to quit smoking? Try this old-time trick: Keep dried cloves in your mouth. Suck on one for a couple of hours, then toss it out and put in a new one. How does it work? The cloves neutralize the taste of nicotine in your mouth, which (according to the experts) is one of the reasons a smoker always wants to reach for another cigarette.

🌿 Make an effective powdered deodorant by mixing equal parts of cornstarch and baking soda with a pinch of ground cloves.

🌿 A great way to ease the pain of a toothache is as close as your spice rack. Put 1 or 2 teaspoons of allspice powder in a cup of boiling water. Steep it for 10 to 20 minutes, and strain it. Gargle with the tea while it's warm, swishing it around your mouth before you spit it out.

🌿 Another quick fix for a toothache is to tuck a clove between the stricken tooth and your cheek. Hold it there for an hour or so, and replace it with a fresh one. If the pain isn't gone after 24 hours, see your dentist.

🍎 Freshen your breath and promote healthy digestion by chewing fennel or dill seeds after meals. (You'll find both kinds of seeds in the spice section of most supermarkets.)

🍎 If you or someone you know has had a poor appetite lately, here's a good remedy: 15 to 30 minutes before every meal, take a mixture of 1 teaspoon of powdered ginger and ½ teaspoon of salt.

🍎 Ease muscle aches and pains by soaking in a bathtub of hot water (as hot as you can stand) with a handful each of dry mustard and sea salt mixed in it. Relax and say *Ahhh…*

🍎 Been chopping onions? Get the odor off of your hands with dry mustard. Just pour a little into your palm, rub it in thoroughly, and rinse it off.

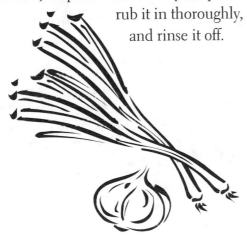

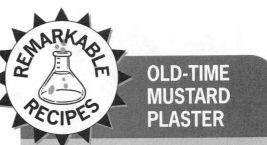

### OLD-TIME MUSTARD PLASTER

Folks used to treat chest colds, flu, and even pneumonia with this remedy. It still works like a charm—but use it with, *not instead of,* your doctor's prescription!

**¼ cup of dry mustard**
**¼ cup of flour**
**3 tbsp. of molasses**
**Thick cream or softened lard**
**Piece of cotton flannel**
**Warm water**

Mix the mustard and flour together, and stir in the molasses. Add enough cream or lard to get an ointment consistency. Dip the cotton flannel in the warm water, wring it out, and lay it on the patient's throat and upper chest, on top of pajamas or a T-shirt, *not against bare skin.* Apply the mustard mixture on top of the the damp cloth, and leave it on for 15 minutes, or until the skin starts to turn red. This stuff is *hot,* so keep close watch and rinse the skin afterwards. If irritation develops, remove the plaster immediately.

## Home Cleaning & Upkeep

◆ Are you cooking up a strong-smelling dinner? Freshen the air by keeping cloves and cinnamon simmering in a pot of water on a back burner.

◆ Getting ready to sell your house? Fifteen minutes or so before the agent arrives with potential buyers, put a handful of dried cloves and a few cinnamon sticks on the stove to simmer, and toss in some grated orange rind. Real estate surveys show that this is one of the two aromas most appealing to potential buyers. (The other is fresh-baked bread.)

◆ To make a strong, but non-toxic drain cleaner, thoroughly mix ½ cup of cream of tartar, 1 cup of salt, and 1 cup of baking soda in a jar with a tight-fitting lid. Pour the mixture into the drain, and follow that up with 2 cups of boiling water. Wait 1 minute, and rinse with cool tap water.

### REMARKABLE RECIPES

### DRY CARPET CLEANER

Don't buy dry carpet cleaner—make your own with this simple recipe.

**2 cups of baking soda**
**½ cup of cornstarch**
**1 tbsp. of ground cloves**
**4–5 crumbled bay leaves**

Mix all of the ingredients together, and store the mixture in a shaker jar. (An empty carpet cleaner can is perfect.) To use the mix, dust the carpet thoroughly with the powder, wait at least 1 hour, and vacuum.

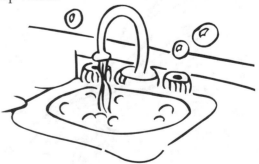

◆ Are your white hankies looking dingy? To bring them back to bright whiteness, soak them for an hour or so in a solution of 1 tablespoon of cream of tartar and 2 teaspoons of laundry detergent in a sinkful of water. Then wash them as usual.

◆ Whipping up a recipe that calls for prepared mustard, and you're fresh out? Use this substitute instead: For every tablespoon of prepared mustard that you need, use ½ teaspoon of dry mustard mixed with 2 teaspoons of vinegar (either white, cider, or wine).

◆ Here's another nose-pleasing trick: Before you vacuum, sprinkle a powdered sweet spice, such as nutmeg or ginger, on the floor. Vacuum it up, then proceed with the rest of the room. You may never buy carpet deodorizer again!

◆ Here's a simple way to freshen up a musty insulated beverage container: Toss 3 or 4 whole dried cloves into it, and let it sit until you need it again. Just be sure that you pour out the cloves before you pour in your coffee or tea! If the taste of cloves doesn't appeal to you, rinse out the container with a mix of baking soda and warm water before you pour in your coffee or tea.

◆ Here's a trick that's been passed down through generations in my family: Keep ants out of the kitchen cupboards by sprinkling some ground cloves all around the perimeter inside the cabinet.

## TRASH TO TREASURE

WHEN YOU finish up all the spice in a jar, don't throw the little thing away! With those perforated tops, spice jars make perfect dispensers for lettuce seeds, carrot seeds, and other tiny seeds that can drive you crazy when you try to sow them by hand. Spice jars are also just the right size for storing leftover seeds. Just combine 1 part seed to 1 part powdered milk, put it in the jar, screw the lid on tight, and store the mixture in the refrigerator (not the freezer) until planting time rolls around.

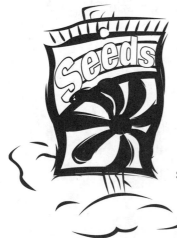

 Yard & Garden

● If you've got an ant invasion on your hands, help is as close as your spice rack—or the supermarket spice section. Just sprinkle cream of tartar, paprika, chili powder, or dried peppermint around the problem areas. Ants find them all disgusting!

● Here's a super-simple way to keep bugs from bugging your garden: Lightly dust your flower and vegetable plants with garlic powder every week or two (and after every rain).

● Protect your plants from powdery mildew and other fungal diseases with this easy-to-make formula: Mix 2 tablespoons of cinnamon powder with 2 cups of rubbing alcohol. Shake well, and let the mixture sit overnight. Filter out the sediment, and pour the liquid into a spray bottle. Spray your plants every week during early spring and during damp spells throughout the growing season.

● To prevent damping-off in your seedlings, use the same formula as above, but substitute hot water for the alcohol, which can dry out the tiny tykes.

# SUGAR

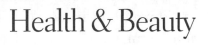

## Health & Beauty

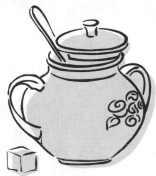

🍎 Got freckles that you're not pleased with? Dissolve a little sugar in 2 tablespoons of lemon juice, then apply the mixture to each freckle with a cotton ball. Repeat the process every couple of days, and the freckles should fade—fast!

🍎 Sugar clears up pimples, too. Just mix it with a few drops of water, and wipe it onto the spots.

🍎 Make an instant granular cleanser by adding a teaspoon of sugar to the cleanser when you wash your face.

🍎 Was your morning coffee a little too hot? Sprinkle a few grains of sugar on your tongue to soothe the burn and speed healing.

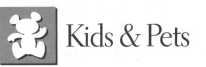

## Kids & Pets

■ Add pizzazz to a birthday cake by substituting sugar cubes for candles. Soak the cubes in vanilla extract (the real stuff, not imitation), and arrange them on the cake. Then, when it's time to launch into "Happy Birthday," light the cubes. They'll sparkle and sputter like tiny sparklers—only better, because the guests can eat them afterwards!

■ Have the kids lost some playing tokens from their favorite board game? Give them sugar cubes to play with instead. Use felt-tip markers or nail polish to give each player's cube a distinguishing mark. The tokens won't survive over the long term, but they'll at least get the youngsters through a round or two.

## REMARKABLE RECIPES

### SWEET SALVE

Sugar helps cuts and scrapes heal much faster, and lessens the risk of infection by helping to keep the wounds dry. So the next time you have a minor mishap, slather on some of this healthful salve.

**4 parts sugar**
**1 part Betadine ointment (available in the supermarket's pharmacy or first-aid section)**

First, wash and dry the wound, and make sure it's stopped bleeding (otherwise, the sugar will make it bleed more). Mix the sugar and Betadine together, dab a thick layer onto the cut, and cover it with a bandage. Repeat the procedure three or four times a day in the beginning, decreasing the applications to once a day as healing progresses.

## Yard & Garden

● Are ants making nuisances of themselves? Mix 2 tablespoons of sugar and 1 tablespoon of baker's yeast in 1 pint of warm water. Then spread the mixture on pieces of cardboard, and set them in the problem areas.

● Here's another ant-busting formula: Mix equal parts of confectioners' sugar and borax with enough water to make a syrup. Pour it into shallow disposable pie pans, and set them where the ants are causing trouble. (Just keep the containers where pets and youngsters can't get at them.)

● When you plant tomatoes, add a spoonful of sugar to each hole. Your tomatoes will be so sweet, you'll want to eat them for dessert!

● Here's a secret for growing the best-tasting rhubarb you've ever had: Several times during the growing season, give it a quality brand of dry, balanced garden food (15-15-15 is good), and mix in ½ cup of sugar per 5 pounds of food. Broadcast this mixture over the planting bed, and water in well.

● Is your garden plagued by nematodes? Kill them off by feeding their sweet tooth. Just till in 5 pounds of sugar for every 50 square feet of planting area. The nematodes will choke on the stuff.

● When you're filling up your lawn mower and some gasoline slops onto the grass, don't panic—you can save that turf. Just mix 6 cups of gypsum with 1 cup of sugar, spread the mixture over the scene of the spill, and water it in well. And next time, remember to fill your mower in the middle of the driveway, not on the lawn!

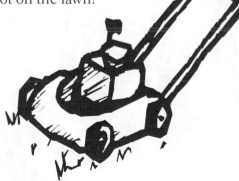

## REMARKABLE RECIPES

### SLUGWEISER

Beer is a classic bait for slug and snail traps, but what attracts the slimy marauders isn't the thought of a good time at the local pub—it's the sugar and yeast in the brew. So don't raid the refrigerator to fill your traps. Use this libation instead.

**1 lb. of brown sugar**
**½ package (1½ tsp.) of dry yeast**
**Warm water**

Pour the sugar and yeast into a 1-gallon container, fill it with warm water, and let it sit for two days, uncovered. Sink some shallow cans into the ground up to their rims, pour in the brew, and watch the culprits belly up to the bar!

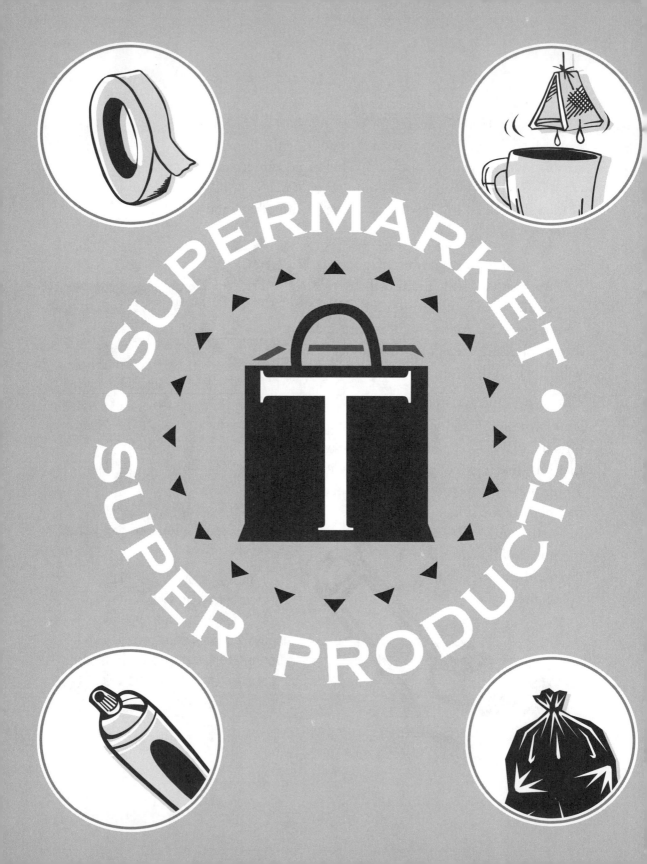

# TAPE

 ## Health & Beauty

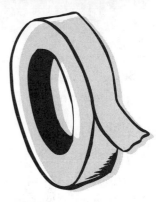

🍎 Coax a splinter out of your skin by covering the spot with tape; any kind will do. It will draw the particle to the surface, and quite possibly, all the way out.

🍎 Here's how to trim bangs as evenly as any pro. When your hair is wet, run transparent tape across your forehead, with the top edge where you want the bottom of your bangs to be. Looking in a mirror, cut just above the tape. You'll have a beauty-shop look without the salon price tag!

🍎 Not sure what shade of fingernail polish you want to wear this evening? Experiment by covering a nail or two with transparent tape and painting the polish over it.

## Home Cleaning & Upkeep

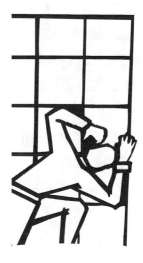

◆ When a plastic tile falls off a wall and you need a quick, but temporary fix, use double-sided tape. Just put a strip along each side of the tile and one in the middle, remove the paper backing from the tape, and push the tile into place. (Note: Use a premium brand for this repair.)

◆ To remove lint or pet hair from upholstery, wrap wide tape, such as masking or mailing tape, around your hand, sticky side out, and press it against the furniture.

# T
## TAPE

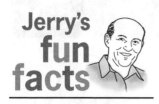
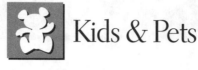 Kids & Pets

■ If the youngsters around your house like to draw with chalk—either indoors on a board or outside on the sidewalk—here's a trick you should know: Wrap one end of the chalk with masking tape to make a child-sized handgrip. That way, the kids can get a firmer grasp, their hands will stay cleaner, and if the chalk drops in the house, there will be less mess to clean up.

■ Keep small children from pushing things into electrical outlets by covering the openings with transparent packing tape (from the supermarket stationery section).

■ Have the kids played their favorite board game so many times that the board's falling apart in the middle? Don't run out and buy a new game just yet. Instead, flip the board over, and run a length of sturdy tape along the fold line. Then, for good measure, cover the front with a sheet of clear Con-Tact® paper. And let the game begin!

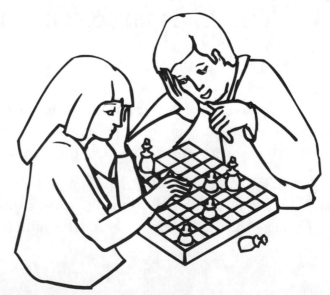

## Workshop & Garage

▼ Getting ready to paint? Before you pour the paint from the can into another container, cover the rim of the can with masking tape. When you're through, simply strip off the tape. The rim will be as clean as new, and you can easily push the lid on tight.

▼ Before you start dismantling anything that has a lot of teeny-tiny parts, spread a length of wide, double-sided tape on your workbench. Then, as you remove each little piece from its home, stick it on the tape. The pieces will stay right there until you're ready to put the appliance (or whatever) back together again.

▼ Make your sandpaper last longer by reinforcing the back with masking tape.

▼ Do plywood sheets splinter when you saw them by hand? This simple maneuver will give you a better chance at a neat, clean cut: Just press a length of masking tape to the underside of the board, along the cutting line, before you start to cut.

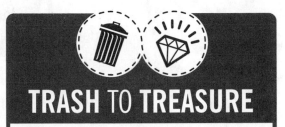

## TRASH TO TREASURE

**SUPERMARKETS CARRY** more kinds of tape than you can shake a shopping list at, but all of them have a sturdy inner reel that's almost as useful as the tape itself. Here are a few things you can do:

○ **Chase birds away from your fruit.** Wrap aluminum foil around them, attach a string, and hang them in your fruit trees and berry bushes.

○ **Make Christmas tree ornaments.** Paint them or cover them with pretty paper, and add a ribbon for hanging.

○ **Store rubber bands.** Dismantle those elastic "nests" in the junk drawer, and snap the bands around a wide tape reel.

○ **Play ring-toss.** Sink a dowel or stick into the ground, and use some empty masking tape reels as the rings.

○ **Make dollhouse furniture.** Cover tape reels with fabric or Con-Tact® paper and, depending on the size, you've got instant dining tables, end tables, nightstands, or ottomans.

▼ Cover the labels on your hardware containers with transparent tape. The labels will be protected from grease, water, and grimy hands, and the writing will stay clear and readable. And that means no more games of "which bin has the finishing nails?"!

▼ Here's one of my favorite quick fixes: Make an ultra-slim saw by wrapping duct tape or electrical tape around one end of a hacksaw blade to form a "handle." This little saw is just the ticket for cutting things that are in really tight spaces, or for loosening windows that have been painted shut.

## Yard & Garden

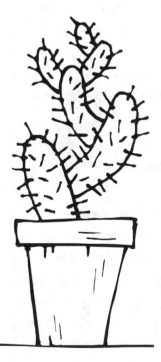

● Are ants farming aphids up in your trees? Clear them out this way: First, blast the aphids off with a strong spray from the garden hose. (If that doesn't do the trick, use the simple soap spray on page 94.) Then, to keep the ants from starting over, wrap double-sided masking tape around the tree trunk. The tape won't harm the tree, but it will trap the ants as they try to scamper up the trunk.

● Do you need to work with a prickly plant like a cactus or a thorny rose? Before you put your gloves on, wrap a piece of heavy tape around each finger. That way, even if the stickers penetrate the gloves, they won't jab your skin. (Duct tape, fabric tape, or electrical tape will give you the surest protection. In a pinch, though, several layers of transparent tape will do the job.)

# TEA

 ## Health & Beauty

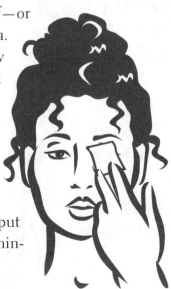

● To soothe the pain of sunburn or other minor burns, soak cotton pads in cold, strong black tea, and apply them to your skin every 10 to 15 minutes until the pain subsides.

● Make tea part of your cancer-prevention plan. Recent research shows that tea is more than a soothing beverage—it actually contains more antioxidants than any fruit or vegetable. Tests have shown that one of its richest compounds, epigallocatechin-3gallate (EGCG, for short), blocks the action of urokinase, an enzyme that cancer cells need so they can attack healthy tissue. So drink up!

● Feel a cold coming on? Fend it off—or at least lessen its severity—by drinking a cup of tea. Research indicates that tea's antioxidants may rev up your immune system and help it fight back when trouble strikes.

● When your eyes are tired and puffy, whether the cause is an allergy or too many hours at the computer, it's tea time. Squeeze most of the moisture out of two used, cooled tea bags, lie down in a comfortable spot, put one bag over each eye, and relax. In 10 to 15 minutes, the swelling should be gone.

# T
## TEA

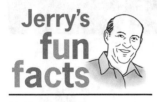
◉ Heal a painful plantar wart by holding a hot, wet teabag on it for 15 minutes every day until the wart shrinks away.

◉ Are your feet, um, aromatic? Try this deodorizing brew: Boil 1 quart of water, add 4 or 5 tea bags, let them steep for 5 to 10 minutes, and remove the bags. When the tea has cooled, pour it into a dishpan or basin, soak your feet in it for about 30 minutes, and dry them without rinsing.

## Home Cleaning & Upkeep

◆ Dye natural-fiber fabric or yarn by soaking it in hot, strong tea. Wait until the material is a shade darker than you want, because it will lighten as it dries. Rinse it in clear, cold water, and let it air dry.

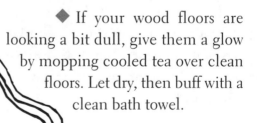

◆ If your wood floors are looking a bit dull, give them a glow by mopping cooled tea over clean floors. Let dry, then buff with a clean bath towel.

◆ Make varnished woodwork shiny-bright by wiping it with a soft cloth dipped in cold tea. Rinse with cool water, and dry with another soft, clean cloth.

◆ Have your black cotton T-shirts taken on a brownish tinge from repeated washings? The next time you wash them, add a cup of strong tea to the rinse water. Those shirts will come out so black that even Zorro would be proud to wear them!

◆ Use instant tea to repair scratches in wood floors or furniture. Just mix 1 teaspoon of instant tea granules with 2 teaspoons of water, dip a cotton swab in the mixture, and apply it to the marks.

◆ Do you want to make some new, white lace curtains, doilies, or table linens match the family heirlooms that your grandma left you? Just steep 6 tea bags per quart of boiling water for 20 minutes. Remove the tea bags, let the tea cool a bit, put your material in the brew, and let it soak for 10 minutes. Wring it out, hang it up to dry, and presto—instant antiques!

◆ You can gently remove a buildup of polish on your wood furniture with brewed tea. Steep two teabags in 4 cups of boiling water and let cool. Dunk a soft, clean cloth in the cooled tea, and wring it out. Then wipe down the furniture.

## TRASH TO TREASURE

**DON'T THROW** away your leftover tea leaves! Instead, save them to make homemade cleansers. Here's how: Mix 1 cup of black tea leaves, 1 teaspoon of baking soda, and a few drops of dishwashing liquid. Then...

○ Use the stuff as you would any scouring powder for general, everyday cleaning.

○ To clean your oven, heat the mixture, and wipe it all over your oven. Let it sit for a few minutes, scrub with a brush or sponge, and rinse with warm water.

○ For pans that are caked with burned-on food, put the mixture inside, and heat it. Remove the pan from the heat, wipe the mixture over the surface, and let it sit for a few minutes. Scrub with a scouring sponge, pour the cleanser out, and wash the pan.

○ Add a squirt of lemon juice to the mix and use to wipe down the inside of your microwave oven.

## ROSE START-UP TONIC

Here's the perfect meal to get your bushes off to a rosy new beginning.

½ gal. of warm tea
1 tbsp. of dishwashing liquid
1 tbsp. of hydrogen peroxide
1 tsp. of whiskey
1 tsp. of Vitamin B₁ Plant Starter

Mix all of these ingredients together in a watering can. Then pour the liquid all around the root zone of each newly planted (or transplanted) rose bush.

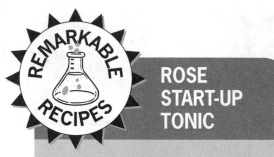

# Yard & Garden

● To protect your onions and radishes from maggots, work tea leaves or tea bags into the soil before you sow your seeds or plant your sets. (Don't worry about the paper tags on the tea bags—they'll break down in a flash.)

● Before you sow any kind of flower or vegetable seeds, soak them in the refrigerator for 24 hours in a solution made of 1 quart of weak tea and 1 teaspoon each of baby shampoo and Epsom salts. This will make the seeds germinate better and faster.

● Once you've sown your seeds, give them an energy boost with this elixir: Mix 1 teaspoon each of bourbon, ammonia, and dishwashing liquid in 1 quart of weak tea. Pour the solution into a hand-held spray bottle, shake it gently, and mist-spray the surface of newly planted seed beds or containers.

● Use cool tea to water acid-loving plants like strawberries, blueberries, azaleas, and rhododendrons.

# TOOTHPASTE

 ## Health & Beauty

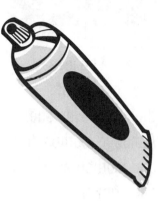

 Dry up pimples by dabbing them with a tiny glob of toothpaste. Let it dry, and rinse with cool water.

 Are itchy mosquito bites driving you nuts? Gently wipe a little bit of toothpaste onto each bite. You'll feel relief fast!

 If you or your kids love to drink grape and other fruit juices, you know how easily they leave stains above your lips. Here's an easy way to "bleach" away juice moustaches: Simply smear a little toothpaste over your upper lip and rinse with clear water. The stain will come off in a hurry, with no scrubbing needed.

## Home Cleaning & Upkeep

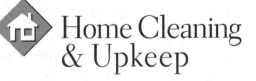

 To get crayon off of painted walls, rub toothpaste onto the marks, then wipe with warm water on a sponge or soft cloth. (This works especially well on white walls.)

 To make a scratched plastic surface look like new again, cover it with toothpaste, using a soft cloth. Wait a minute or two, and buff with a clean, dry cloth.

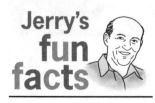

◆ Use toothpaste to polish silver and remove scratches. Squeeze the paste onto a soft cotton cloth, and rub it onto the silver in small circles. Rinse immediately.

◆ Is your gold jewelry looking dingy? Toothpaste will make it bright and shiny again. Just put a tiny glob on a soft cotton cloth, wipe the metal clean, and rinse with clear water.

◆ Clean piano keys with a little toothpaste on a damp cloth. Rub the keys well, wipe dry, and buff with a soft, dry cloth.

◆ Need to remove ink spots or grass stains from fabric? Squeeze toothpaste onto the stains, scrub with a toothbrush, rinse, and launder as usual.

 # Workshop & Garage

▼ Use toothpaste to remove light scratches from your car's windows or mirrors. Just squeeze a little mildly abrasive toothpaste—not the gel kind—onto a soft, cotton flannel cloth, and rub the scratches very lightly until they vanish.

▼ When you need to fill nail holes in a white wall, *fast*, and you're fresh out of spackling compound, use toothpaste instead. It's not a permanent fix, but it will cover the holes until you can do a proper repair job. Just squeeze a dab of white toothpaste onto your finger or a cotton swab, fill the hole, and wipe off the excess with a damp sponge.

# TRASH BAGS

##  Home Cleaning & Upkeep

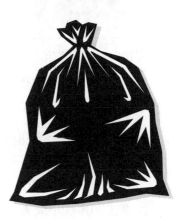

◆ Use a giant lawn-and-leaf trash bag as a waterproof smock for sloppy cleaning chores. Just cut a head-sized hole in the bottom and an arm hole in each side, and slip the bag over your head.

◆ Here's a painless way to battle clutter: Tie the handles of drawstring trash bags to coat hangers, and hang one in each closet in the house. Then, each time you come across a garment that you no longer wear, a toy that the kids no longer play with, or a gadget you haven't used in ages, toss it in the bag. When you've got a bunch of filled bags, you're all set for your blockbuster garage sale—or a trip to the local thrift store.

## 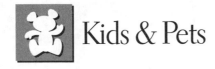 Kids & Pets

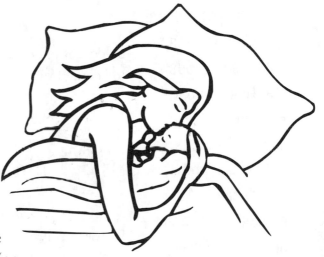

■ When a tyke in diapers comes to spend the night, waterproof a mattress by cutting open a giant trash bag and putting it under the sheet.

■ When you go on the road with a tiny tot, pack a trash bag (or two) to use as an emergency diaper-changing mat.

257

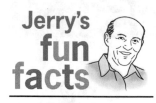

■ Cut trash bags into strips, and use them as waterproof stuffing for pool and tub toys.

■ Are the youngsters having a camp-out in the backyard? Keep their sleeping bags dry by spreading trash bags on the ground underneath them.

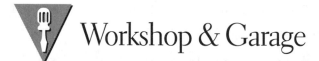

# Workshop & Garage

▼ Before you start a paint job, put trash bags over lamps, ceiling fans, small pieces of furniture, and anything else that your drop cloths don't cover.

▼ Cut head and arm holes in a giant trash bag, and stash it in your car's glove compartment to use as an emergency rain slicker. (Better yet, keep several bags on hand so your passengers can stay dry, too!)

▼ If your car has to stay outdoors overnight in cold weather, cover the windshield with a trash bag or two to keep it free of frost and ice.

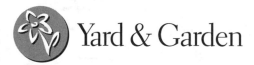

# Yard & Garden

● Use extra-large trash bags as protective covers for your outdoor furniture, bicycles, barbecue grill, or anything else that sits outside and needs protection from the elements.

● Foil Colorado potato beetles with heavy-duty trash bags. Here's how: In fall or very early spring, dig a trench about 8 inches deep around your target plants, with the sides as close to vertical as possible. Then line the trench with trash bags. When the beetles wake up in the spring, they're too weak to fly, so they have to walk to get breakfast. When they reach the trench, they'll fall in and slide around on the plastic until birds eat them.

● Going away on vacation? Here's an easy way to keep your houseplants watered in your absence: Line your bathtub with trash bags, and cover them with a big, wet towel. Set your plants on the towel, and just before you leave, water them thoroughly. Assuming the pots have drainage holes at the bottom, the plants should stay in fine shape for two weeks or so.

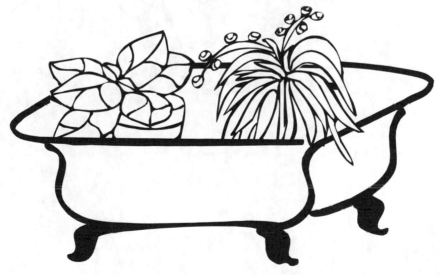

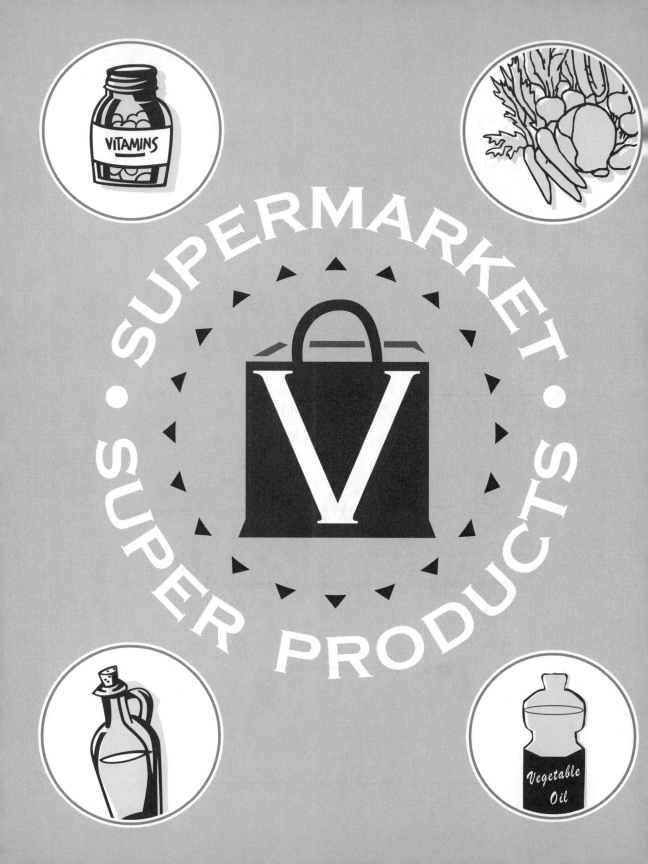

# VEGETABLES

 ## Health & Beauty

Are you suffering from painful hemorrhoids? Try this all-natural cure: Chop up a cabbage, lay the pieces on a towel, and sit on them for 30 minutes or so. Just don't forget to take your pants off first!

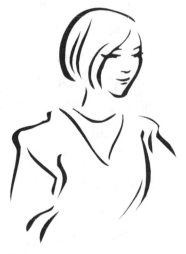

Do you have oily skin? Here's a super-simple way to tone it up: Mash a tomato, and spread it onto your face. Wait about 30 minutes, and then rinse with cool water.

This masque is another neat treat for oily skin: Boil three large carrots until they're soft. Mash them, and add 5 tablespoons of honey. Massage the mixture gently onto your face, using a circular motion, and leave it on for 20 minutes. Rinse with warm water, and pat dry. (Before you use this on your face, test it on an inconspicuous spot, like inside the crook of your arm, to make sure it doesn't turn your skin slightly — but temporarily — orange.)

Got oily hair? Here's a treatment that will get rid of excess oil without drying out your scalp. Chop up three, good-sized raw carrots, and purée them in a blender. Apply the purée to your scalp, and leave it on for 10 to15 minutes. Rinse it off with cool water.

# V

## VEGETABLES

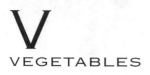

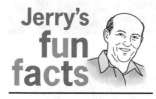

Eggplant might seem like just another mild-mannered vegetable, but it has a long history of being touted with having some pretty impressive powers—both good and bad. Folks in medieval Europe considered it an aphrodisiac. But in the 1800s, doctors in Europe and Southeast Asia blamed the poor eggplant for all sorts of maladies, from epilepsy to cancer. Go figure!

❧ Banish blackheads by rubbing the affected areas with a slice or two of tomato once a day.

❧ Use lettuce to relieve skin rashes and sunburn. Separate and clean the leaves of one small head, toss them into boiling water for 5 minutes, and drain (saving the water). Let the leaves cool, then put them on your face and neck. Wait 5 to 10 minutes if you can—the leaves will be slippery! Pat dry, without rinsing. Store the reserved liquid in a covered container in the refrigerator, and use it as a skin lotion.

## Home Cleaning & Upkeep

◆ Polish your pewter by rubbing it with the outer leaves of a fresh head of cabbage and then buffing with a soft cloth.

◆ To remove an ink spot from any kind of fabric, put a slice of raw tomato on the stain. Wait until the tomato has absorbed the ink, and launder as usual.

◆ Use natural vegetable dyes to color Easter eggs. Put the eggs in a single layer in a pan with just enough water to cover them. Add about 1 teaspoon of vinegar and about 2½ cups of your chosen fruit or vegetable (see Jerry's Fun Facts on page 263). Bring the water to a boil, reduce the heat, and simmer for 15 to 20 minutes. For darker colors, strain the dye into a bowl with the eggs, and let it sit in the refrigerator overnight.

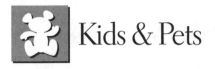

## Kids & Pets

■ Do you need nontoxic paint for your young artists? Then make some vegetable paint. Here's how: Put some veggies in a Crock-Pot® with enough water to barely cover them, and let it cook all night. Strain out the solids, and you've got paint (see Jerry's Fun Facts, at right). Or, if your creative tots are more into writing than drawing, they can use the stuff as colorful ink.

■ Is there a teething puppy in the house? Give him a crunchy raw carrot to chew on. It'll soothe his gums—and save your slippers.

■ Many raw vegetables make great, healthy treats for dogs of any age. The menu includes broccoli, baby carrots, cauliflower, green beans, tomatoes, and zucchini.

■ Could your pooch stand to lose a few pounds? This two-step weight-reduction plan beats diet dog foods, paws down. **Step 1:** Cut back on the daily ration of dog food and make up the difference with cooked vegetables. (Caution: Be wary of corn, which triggers allergies in many dogs. And avoid onions, which can cause fever, vomiting, and diarrhea.) **Step 2:** Go for a 2-mile-long walk together every day—it'll put both of you in better shape!

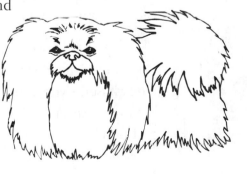

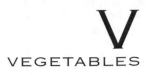

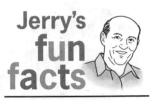

### Jerry's fun facts

The supermarket is full of vegetables and fruits that you can use to make paint, ink, or Easter egg dye. Here's a rundown:

*Red:* Fresh beets or cranberries, frozen raspberries, red onion skins

*Orange:* Yellow onion skins

*Yellow:* Carrot tops (the green part), orange or lemon peels

*Pale green:* Spinach

*Green-gold:* Golden Delicious apple peels

*Blue:* Red cabbage leaves or canned blueberries

# V

VEGETABLES

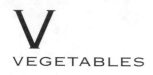

## BRUSSELS SPROUTS ELIXIR

If you're looking for a nontoxic herbicide for annual weeds, this recipe's for you. Serve it up in early spring, before the seeds germinate. (The secret ingredient is in the Brussels sprouts—it's thiocyanate, a chemical that's toxic to newly germinated seeds, especially small ones.)

**2 cups of Brussels sprouts**
**Water**
**½ tsp. of dishwashing liquid**

In a blender or food processor, blend the Brussels sprouts with just enough water to make a thick mush. Add ½ teaspoon of dishwashing liquid, and pour the mixture into cracks in your sidewalk or driveway, or anyplace you want to stop weeds before they germinate. (Just be careful where you use this stuff: Although thiocyanate won't hurt established plants, it can't tell the difference between the seeds you've sown—or the volunteers you're hoping for—and the weeds you want to get rid of!)

 Yard & Garden

● To trap slugs or snails, slice some cabbage or lettuce leaves into thin strips, and put them in a shallow cat food or tuna can filled with salt water. The slugs will home in on the cabbage, fall into the drink, and drown.

● Don't have any cans on hand to make the traps in the tip above? Just set whole cabbage or lettuce leaves on the ground near your slug-infested plants. The slimers will crawl under them during the heat of the day, and you can scoop them up and drop them into a bucket of salt water.

● Rid your garden of wireworms with this trick: Punch medium-sized nail holes into the sides of large cans. Fill them about halfway with cut-up carrots, and bury them so that the tops are just above ground. Cover the openings with small boards, and put mulch on top. Once a week, pull up the cans and empty them into a bucket of soapy water. Then, re-bait and re-bury your traps.

● Do you eat a lot of asparagus at your house? If so, you've got a terrific nematode chaser. Every time you boil or steam the yummy spears, pour the cooking water on the ground close to your troubled plants. Nematodes *hate* asparagus juice!

# VEGETABLE OIL

 Health & Beauty

For a soothing, moisturizing bath, warm some vegetable oil, and rub it on your skin. Wait 5 minutes, then ease into the tub and lather up.

Give yourself a hot-oil hair treatment. Rub heated vegetable oil into your scalp, and work it through your hair to the ends. Wait 15 minutes, and shampoo as usual.

Been on your feet all day? Soothe those tired tootsies this way: Rub warmed vegetable oil into the skin, wrap a hot, damp towel around your feet, and relax for 10 minutes. You'll be ready to dance all night!

High-quality vegetable oil is perfect for removing eye makeup. Just rub on a thick coat with your finger, leave the oil in place for about a minute to dissolve the makeup, and then wipe it off with a cotton ball.

Keep cuticles moisturized by massaging vegetable oil around the base of each nail.

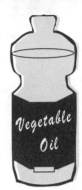

**REMARKABLE RECIPES**

## HOMEMADE COLD CREAM

You *could* go out and pay a lot of money for a fancy cold cream. Or you could make your own!

**1 egg yolk**
**2 tbsp. of lemon juice**
**½ cup of light vegetable oil**
**½ cup of olive oil**

Combine the egg yolk and lemon juice, and mix with a wire whisk. Gradually add the oils, continuing to stir, until the mixture thickens. If it's too thick, add more lemon juice; if it's too thin, add a little more egg yolk. Store in a covered container in the refrigerator.

265

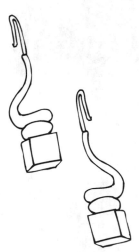

🍎 Want a simple, homemade bubble bath? Put 2 cups of vegetable oil, 3 tablespoons of mild shampoo, and ¼ teaspoon of your favorite perfume or scented oil in a blender. Blend at high speed, and store in a capped bottle at room temperature. At bath time, pour about ¼ cup of the mixture under running water.

🍎 Earrings being stubborn again? They'll glide right in if you rub them and your earlobes with a little vegetable oil.

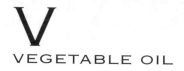

## Home Cleaning & Upkeep

◆ This trick will make wooden cutting boards and salad bowls last almost indefinitely: Every few months, wipe a thick coat of vegetable oil onto the wood, let it sit overnight, and wipe off the excess. This also works great on butcher block table tops.

◆ Use vegetable oil to lubricate things like squeaky door hinges, stiff locks, and stuck window gliders.

◆ Got some leather gloves that have turned as stiff as boards? Rub a little vegetable oil into them. They'll be as soft as new in no time!

◆ To make an instant oil lamp, pour vegetable oil into a metal or heat-proof ceramic bowl, and insert a cotton wick (available at craft stores).

◆ Looking for a top-notch furniture polish for your treasured antiques? Look no further—here it is: Just combine 1 cup of vegetable oil with ½ cup of lemon juice. Massage it into the wood with a soft, clean cotton cloth, and buff with a second clean cloth.

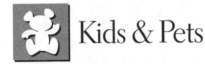

## Kids & Pets

■ Did some young model builders get glue on the dining table? Rub the wood with a little vegetable oil on a soft cotton cloth. The glue will come right out.

■ Prevent hair balls from forming in Puffy's tummy by mixing 1 teaspoon of vegetable oil into her food once a week.

■ Does your cat have ear mites? Clear them out this way: Put a few drops of vegetable oil into the ear, and massage it gently. Then clean out all of the debris with a cotton ball or swab. Repeat in each ear once a day for three days, and the mites should be gone. If they're not, or if kitty still shows signs of discomfort, call your vet.

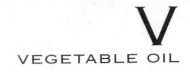

**REMARKABLE RECIPES**

## BATHTUB COOKIES

These fun, bath-time "cookies" are the perfect bribe for reluctant young bathers. They also make great gifts.

**2 cups of fine-grain sea salt***
**½ cup of cornstarch**
**½ cup of baking soda**
**2 tbsp. of light vegetable oil**
**1 tsp. of vitamin E oil**
**6 drops of your favorite scented oil**
**6 drops of food coloring (optional)**

Mix all of the ingredients together, roll out the dough, and cut out shapes with cookie cutters. Bake at 350°F for 10 to 12 minutes. (Don't overbake!) Let the cookies cool completely, and put them in a big glass jar or other decorative container. To use, just add one or two cookies to the bathwater, and enjoy!

*If your supermarket doesn't have fine-grain sea salt, use Kosher salt instead, and run it through your blender or coffee grinder.*

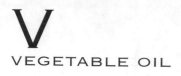
■ No matter how your pooch managed to get burrs, tar, or some other mysterious, sticky stuff in his hair, this gentle process will get it out in no time: Saturate the problem area with vegetable oil, and work it into the hair and skin. Then wash with a good dog shampoo, rinse immediately, and brush.

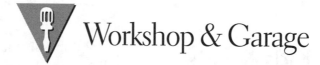

## Workshop & Garage

▼ Keep your tools free of rust and corrosion by giving them a good cleaning, and lightly coating all of the metal surfaces with vegetable oil.

▼ Got some oil-based paint on your skin? Don't use turpentine or other harsh solvents to get it off; reach for the vegetable oil instead. Just wipe a generous amount of oil on with a soft cloth or paper towel, and rub. Then wash with warm, soapy water, and dry off thoroughly.

▼ Do you live in an area where winter gets so cold that your car doors freeze shut? End that frustration by rubbing the gaskets with vegetable oil before the weather gets bad. It will seal out water without harming the gaskets.

Yard & Garden

● Has pruning evergreens left you with sap all over your hands? Rub them with vegetable oil, and wipe with a paper towel. Your skin will soon be sap-free.

● Keep your pruning shears working smoothly by dribbling a little vegetable oil into the pivot point after every use.

● When mosquito season rolls around, and you've got puddles of standing water that you can't drain, how do you keep them from turning into skeeter maternity wards? Simple: Pour a thin layer of vegetable oil onto the water. The oil will smother any newly hatched eggs.

● Have your plants broken out in rust? After you've removed and destroyed the badly infected leaves, nix any lingering fungus with this formula: Mix 6 tablespoons of vegetable oil and 2 tablespoons each of baking soda and kelp extract in 1 gallon of water. Pour the solution into a hand-held sprayer, and spray the foliage from top to bottom. Repeat every week to 10 days during damp or humid weather.

## REMARKABLE RECIPES

### BASIC OIL MIXTURE

Scale insects and a whole lot of other pests go belly-up when they strike oil—or rather, when oil strikes *them*!

**1 cup of vegetable oil**
**1 tbsp. of Murphy's Oil Soap®**

Pour the oil and the oil soap into a plastic squeeze bottle, and store it at room temperature. To use it, put 1 tablespoon of the mixture in 2 cups of water in a hand-held spray bottle, and spray your pest-ridden plants from top to bottom. (Shake the bottle now and then to make sure the oil and water stay mixed.)

# V

# VINEGAR

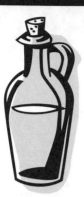

## ✚ Health & Beauty

🍎 Before you polish your nails, wipe them with a cotton ball dipped in vinegar to get rid of any oil and dirt—thereby making the polish adhere better and last longer, for a perfect manicure.

🍎 Has residue from shampoos and conditioners left your scalp flaky and irritated? Here's a simple remedy: Rinse your hair with a solution of 3 tablespoons of white vinegar in a cup of warm water. Work it in well, and follow with a clear water rinse until the vinegar is gone.

🍎 Planning on spending some time in the sun? Put some white vinegar in a spray bottle and keep it in the refrigerator. Then, if you stay out too long and wind up with a sunburn, spritz yourself with the vinegar to cool and soothe your skin. (This trick also works well for soothing minor burns from the stove or a hot iron.)

🍎 If you work out at a gym or health club, this tip's for you: Keep a spray bottle of vinegar in your tote bag or locker, and use it to kill the fungus that causes athlete's foot. Each time you get out of the shower, spray your toes thoroughly, rinse them with clear water, and dry them well.

🍎 Use herbal vinegar as a skin cleanser, toner, and astringent (see Easy Herbal Vinegar, at right).

🍎 Pat white vinegar on insect bites to ease the pain and itch.

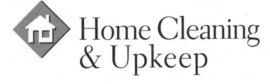 Home Cleaning & Upkeep

◆ Are your windows really greasy? Then wash them with a solution of ½ cup of white vinegar and 2 tablespoons of lemon juice (either fresh or bottled) in 1 quart of warm water. It works like a charm every time!

◆ Want to turn dull metal furniture bright and shiny again? Spray it with a solution made of equal parts of vinegar and water, and rub with a sponge or nylon scrub pad. There's no need to rinse before toweling it dry.

◆ Is the showerhead clogged again? Unscrew it, and soak it in a solution of equal parts of vinegar and warm water for 15 minutes or so. Your shower will flow like Niagara Falls!

**REMARKABLE RECIPES**

## EASY HERBAL VINEGAR

Just about anything that plain vinegar can do, herbal vinegar can do better! Besides adding pizzazz to any recipe, it's like a combination first-aid kit and beauty spa in a bottle. And it couldn't be easier to make! Here's the basic recipe.

**½ cup of dried herbs, or 1 cup of fresh herb leaves (washed and dried)**
**2 cups of white vinegar**

Put the herbs in a sterilized glass jar, and mash them slightly with a spoon. Pour the vinegar over the herbs, cover the jar tightly, and let the mixture steep in a dark place at room temperature for one to three weeks. Shake the jar every few days, and taste the vinegar once a week until the flavor reaches the desired intensity. Add more herbs if you need to. When the flavor suits you, strain out the solids, and pour the vinegar into a sterilized bottle with a tight cap. Keep it away from direct light, which can rapidly decrease the herbs' potency.

◆ Here are some ideas for herbs to use in your homemade vinegar (see Easy Herbal Vinegar on page 271): **Bay leaves:** antiseptic; freshens all types of skin. **Marjoram or oregano:** antiseptic; soothes sore throats; relieves aching joints and muscles. **Mint:** relieves headaches; cools and refreshes; good for normal skin. **Parsley:** cleanses and balances oily skin; lightens freckles; adds shine to dark hair. **Rosemary:** antiseptic; repels insects; good for oily skin. **Thyme:** antiseptic; deodorizes.

◆ This is a noisy way to clean your garbage disposal, but it works like a dream: Fill a couple of ice cube trays with vinegar (any kind will do) and freeze them. Run the cubes through the disposal, and let the cold water run for a minute or so. The grinding of ice on the blades will remove any clinging food particles, and the vinegar will eliminate odors.

◆ When you wash a plastic shower curtain or tablecloth, add a cup of vinegar to the rinse water. The plastic will dry soft and supple.

◆ Have your old pantyhose gotten baggy? To get them back into shape, soak them for 15 minutes in a sinkful of water with 2 teaspoons of vinegar added to it. Rinse in clear water, hang the hose up to dry, and they'll be as good as new!

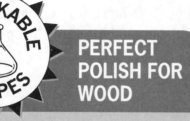

**REMARKABLE RECIPES**

## PERFECT POLISH FOR WOOD

Here's a great furniture polish for any kind of wood furniture.

**½ cup of linseed oil**
**¼ cup of malt vinegar**
**1 tsp. of lemon or lavender oil**

Put the linseed oil and vinegar in a clean jar with a tight lid, and shake it vigorously. Stir in the lemon or lavender oil. Apply it to your furniture with a clean, soft cotton cloth, and buff with a second, clean cloth. (In hot, humid weather, reverse the proportions, so that you're combining ¼ cup of linseed oil and ½ cup of vinegar, because damp heat tends to make oil, well, oilier.)

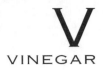

◆ Going away for a while? Leave a small, open container of vinegar in each room of your house while you're gone. It will keep the air fresh, so you won't come home to that closed-up smell.

◆ Want to keep your new blue jeans from fading? Before you wash them for the first time, soak them for an hour in a solution of ½ cup of vinegar and 2 quarts of water.

◆ Whoops! You accidentally put too much laundry detergent in the washing machine. Now what? Just add 2 tablespoons of vinegar to the water to counteract the extra detergent.

◆ Here's an easy, natural way to sweeten and freshen any load of laundry: Just add ½ cup of baking soda to the wash cycle, and ½ cup of white vinegar to the rinse cycle. (Use a little more of each if you have hard water. The exact amount you need will vary, depending on your water's mineral content.)

◆ Polish patent leather shoes, purses, and belts by wiping them with a little vinegar on a clean, soft cloth. Wipe the surface dry with another soft cloth.

◆ Wash your washing machine every now and then by filling it with warm water and about ½ cup of vinegar (but no clothes!), and then running it through a complete cycle.

◆ Has soap scum built up on your glassware? Run the pieces through the dishwasher, using ½ cup of bleach in the wash cycle and ½ cup of vinegar in the rinse phase.

# V
## VINEGAR

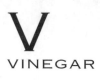

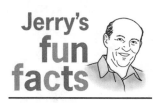
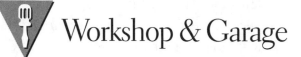

## Workshop & Garage

▼ When you have to leave your car outdoors overnight in the winter, keep the windows free of frost and ice with this simple trick: Spray the outside of the windows with a solution made of 3 parts vinegar to 1 part water.

▼ To clean the inside of your car from stem to stern—including glass, chrome, vinyl, rubber, and even leather—use a spray made of equal parts of vinegar and water, and wipe with a clean, soft cloth.

▼ Got an unpleasant odor in your car? Make it fade fast by pouring a little vinegar into a shallow bowl and leaving it in the car overnight. Just remember to take the dish out before you go for a spin, or you'll wind up with a car that smells like salad dressing!

▼ To remove a stubborn bumper sticker, coat it with vinegar, wait until the liquid has thoroughly penetrated the paper, and scrape it away with a plastic scraper.

▼ Uh, oh! You forgot to clean your paintbrushes yesterday, and now they're stiff and hard. They'll be as clean and soft as new if you do this: Pour enough vinegar into a saucepan to cover the bristles. Heat it to a simmer, put the brushes in the pan, and keep them in the simmering liquid until the bristles soften up. Wash the brushes as usual, and put them away until it's time to paint again.

▼ Banish rust from tools or hardware by soaking the pieces overnight in full-strength vinegar. The rust will dissolve like magic.

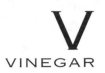

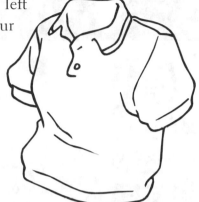

▼ Has your latest workshop project left you with more glue on your shirt than on your fabulous creation? Don't worry—just put 3 tablespoons of vinegar in a sinkful of warm water, and soak the shirt until the glue has dissolved.

 Yard & Garden

● Extend the life of cut flowers by adding 2 tablespoons of white vinegar and 2 tablespoons of white sugar per quart of water.

● Do you want to lower your soil's pH to please acid-loving plants like azaleas, camellias, or blueberries? Vinegar could be your answer. Every three months during the growing season, mix 2 cups of distilled vinegar per 2 gallons of water, and pour the solution on the ground around each plant's drip line.

● Slugs driving you crazy? Shortly after dark, fill a spray bottle with a half-and-half solution of vinegar and water, head out to the garden, and let 'em have it. Or pour the solution into squirt guns, put a bounty on the slugs' heads, and send a posse of neighborhood youngsters out to do the job!

**REMARKABLE RECIPES**

### SEED SEND-OFF

When you start your seeds—indoors or out—give them this nourishing soak to start 'em out strong.

**1 cup of white vinegar**
**1 tbsp. of baby shampoo or dishwashing liquid**
**2 cups of warm water**

Mix the vinegar and baby shampoo or dishwashing liquid in the warm water. Soak your seeds in the solution overnight before planting them in well-prepared soil.

# V

# VITAMINS

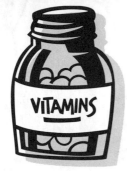 Health & Beauty

🍎 Nourish and soften your face with this sweet-smelling masque. In a bowl, mix 2 drops of vitamin E oil, 2 tablespoons of mashed strawberries, and 1 tablespoon each of coconut oil, olive oil, and light vegetable oil. Smooth the mixture sparingly onto your face, and go about your business for a few hours. Then rinse with warm water, and pat your face with witch hazel on a cotton pad. (Store the leftover moisturizer in a covered container in the refrigerator, and use within a week.)

🍎 Looking for a good, whole-body moisturizer? They don't come any better—or simpler—than this one: As soon as you get out of the shower, *before* you dry off, slather yourself with vitamin E oil. It will trap moisture against your skin, and leave you feeling baby-soft all over—guaranteed!

🍎 If you've been spending more time than usual in the great outdoors, treat yourself to this rejuvenating facial: Drain the contents of five vitamin E capsules into a small bowl, and add 2 teaspoons of plain yogurt and ½ teaspoon each of honey and lemon juice. Mix well, and apply it to your face with a cotton ball. Wait about 10 minutes, and rinse with warm water.

🍎 Ease the itch of dry skin patches by rubbing on a generous amount of vitamin E oil after you bathe.

🍎 Do you have a scar that's more prominent than you'd like? Minimize its appearance by rubbing a few drops of vitamin E oil into it daily.

🍎 For an ultra-simple *and* ultra-softening bath, mix the contents of 5 or 6 vitamin E capsules with 1 or 2 tablespoons of your favorite fragrance oil, and pour it under running water in the tub.

🍎 If you like to sport a summer tan, this lotion's for you. In a blender, mix the juice of 1 lemon with ¼ cup each of strong black tea and salt-free mayonnaise. Pour the mixture into a lidded container, squeeze the contents of 5 vitamin E capsules (400 IU each) into it, and stir. Keep the lotion in the refrigerator, and slather it on before you head out to bask in the sun. Just don't stay too long!

🍎 No skin cream can turn back the clock, but this simple treatment *will* make your face look younger, at least for a while. Just mash a peeled, medium-sized banana and mix it with ¼ cup of heavy whipping cream. Stir in the contents of 1 vitamin E capsule. Smooth the concoction onto your face and neck, wait 10 to 15 minutes, and wipe it off with a damp washcloth.

**REMARKABLE RECIPES**

## CHOCOLATE LIP BALM

When harsh winter air leaves your lips cracked and dry—and you need a sweet treat to get you through the cold, dark days—reach for this recipe. And while you're at it, make a few extras as gifts for all the choc-aholics in your life!

**2 tbsp. of petroleum jelly**
**1 tbsp. of powdered chocolate milk mix (or to taste)\***
**1 vitamin E capsule**

Put the petroleum jelly into a microwave-safe container, and nuke it at 30-second intervals until the jelly is melted. (Be patient—it might take several minutes or more.) Snip open the capsule and pour the vitamin E oil into the melted petroleum jelly, and then stir. Mix in the chocolate milk powder, return it to the microwave for another 30 seconds, and mix again until smooth. Let the mixture cool, and pour it into small, clean, airtight containers.

*\* Or substitute vanilla- or strawberry-flavored milk mix.*

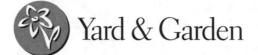

## Yard & Garden

● Getting ready to plant bare-root roses? Ease them into their new home by soaking the roots for 24 hours in this solution: 1 vitamin $B_1$ tablet dissolved in a little hot water, 1 tablespoon of Epsom salts, and 1 teaspoon of baby shampoo per gallon of water.

● Are your houseplants looking less than chipper? The problem could be that they're getting too much food all at once. Instead of feeding and watering them separately, add 10 percent of the recommended dose of your regular plant food to the watering can each time you give them a drink, and mix in this kicker: one vitamin $B_1$ tablet dissolved in hot water, ½ tablespoon of unflavored gelatin, 1 ounce of hydrogen peroxide, and 1 capful of whiskey.

● To keep your Christmas tree looking festive all through the holiday season, follow this routine: Before you put it into its stand, cut 1 inch off the bottom of the trunk, and soak it overnight in a bucket of very warm water with four multivitamin tablets with iron, 2 cups of clear corn syrup, and 2 tablespoons of bleach. And once you've set it up, make sure you keep plenty of water in the stand at all times!

● Help stem cuttings form roots faster by giving them doses of vitamin $B_1$. For future plants being started in water, add ½ tablet per 8-ounce glass. If you're using a commercial starting mix, use 1 tablet per quart each time you water your cuttings. (Either way, dissolve the vitamin tablet in hot water first.)

# VODKA & GIN

 ## Health & Beauty

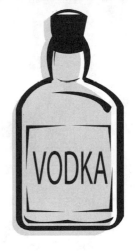

🍎 Here's a simple alternative to aerosol hair sprays: Just peel and chop two lemons, and put them into 2 cups of boiling water. Let the mix simmer until the fruit is tender, cool it, and strain it into a spray bottle. Add 1 tablespoon of vodka, and shake well. If the potion is too sticky, dilute it with a little water.

🍎 Looking for a new brand of mouthwash? Don't buy it! Make your own instead with this simple formula: Put ¾ cup of vodka and 20 drops of lemon juice in a bottle with a tight cap, shake well, and let it sit for one week at room temperature. To use it, mix 1 part solution with 2 parts distilled water, and gargle.

🍎 To make your hair shine like the sun, mix equal parts of vodka and your regular shampoo before each washing.

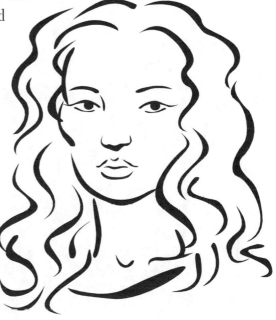

🍎 If you prefer your mouthwash on the spicy side, try this potion instead: Mix ¼ cup of vodka, ¼ cup of water, and 5 drops each of clove, orange, and cinnamon oil. Store the solution in a dark-colored glass bottle with a spray top. Shake well before using it.

# V

## VODKA & GIN

🍎 Before cold and flu season starts, arm yourself with this tonic: Mix ¾ cup of vodka, ¾ cup of distilled water, and 2½ tablespoons of dried echinacea root (from the health-food section of your supermarket) in a glass jar. Stir to blend. Store it in a cool, dark place for two weeks, and strain the tincture into glass bottles with tight-fitting caps. Then, at the first sign of cold or flu symptoms, mix 2 or 3 drops in a glass of water, and drink to your health!

🍎 Tired of your old deodorant? Try this simple alternative: Fill a large, clean, wide-mouth canning jar with grass clippings from a lawn that has *not* been treated with chemical pesticides or fertilizers. Cover the clippings with vodka, close the jar tightly, put it in a cool, dark place for 7 to 10 days, and shake it now and then. Strain out the clippings, and pour the liquid into a bottle. (An old, clean roll-on deodorant bottle is perfect.) If you don't have a roll-on bottle, apply with your fingertips.

🍎 Do you need *fast* sunburn relief? Use plain old gin. Just pour it into a spray bottle, and spritz your sore skin. Follow up with a moisturizing lotion.

🍎 Soak away the pain of sunburn by adding 1 or 2 cups of gin to tepid bath water. Be sure to use a good moisturizer after you gently pat yourself dry.

## REMARKABLE RECIPES

### BAY RUM AFTERSHAVE

If you're looking for a homemade gift idea for the men in your life, you've come to the right place. This classic potion is the perfect answer—especially for those guys who have everything!

**½ cup of vodka**
**2 tbsp. of dark rum**
**2 dried bay leaves**
**¼ tsp. of allspice**
**1 cinnamon stick**
**Rind from 1 small orange,**
  **shredded**

Mix all of the ingredients together. Pour the mixture into a clean jar with a tight lid, and set it in a cool, dark place for two weeks. Strain out the solids, and pour the liquid into a nice-looking bottle. Add a label, if you'd like. That's all there is to it!

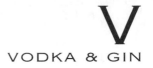

🍎 Are you troubled by arthritis or migraine headaches? Try this recipe for pain relief—a lot of folks swear by it, including radio commentator Paul Harvey. Put a box of golden raisins in a bowl, and add just enough gin to cover them completely. Let them sit, uncovered, at room temperature until there is no standing liquid. Transfer the raisins to a container that you can tightly close, and eat nine of them every day.

##  Home Cleaning & Upkeep

◆ Your upholstery has picked up an unpleasant aroma, and there's no time to get one of those special fabric deodorizers. So what do you do? Reach for the vodka! Mix it half-and-half with water in a spray bottle, and spritz it on the cloth. It works just as well as commercial products on any kind of fiber, it evaporates quickly, and it leaves no tell-tale scent behind. What more could you ask for?

◆ Need to clean a mirror *immediately*, and you're all out of the usual glass cleaners? Use this easy-as-pie tip from a housekeeping book of the early 1800s: Pour a splash of gin on a clean, soft cloth and wipe. It's guaranteed to remove even smoke film and splattered flies!

# V
## VODKA & GIN

 Yard & Garden

● Here's the perfect way to nix those *really* stubborn weeds: Mix 2 tablespoons each of gin, vinegar, and dishwashing liquid per quart of hot water. Pour the solution into a hand-held spray bottle, and blast those weeds to you-know-where!

● Keep your cut flowers fresher longer by adding a shot of vodka to the water in the vase.

● Your flowering houseplants will bloom to beat the band if you give them a dose of this elixir every two weeks or so: Mix ½ tablespoon of vodka, ½ tablespoon of ammonia, ½ tablespoon of hydrogen peroxide, ¼ teaspoon of instant tea granules, and 1 multivitamin tablet with iron into a gallon of warm water. Store in a container with a cap, and use 1 cup of the solution per gallon of water at plant-feeding time. (For non-flowering plants, use bourbon instead of vodka.)

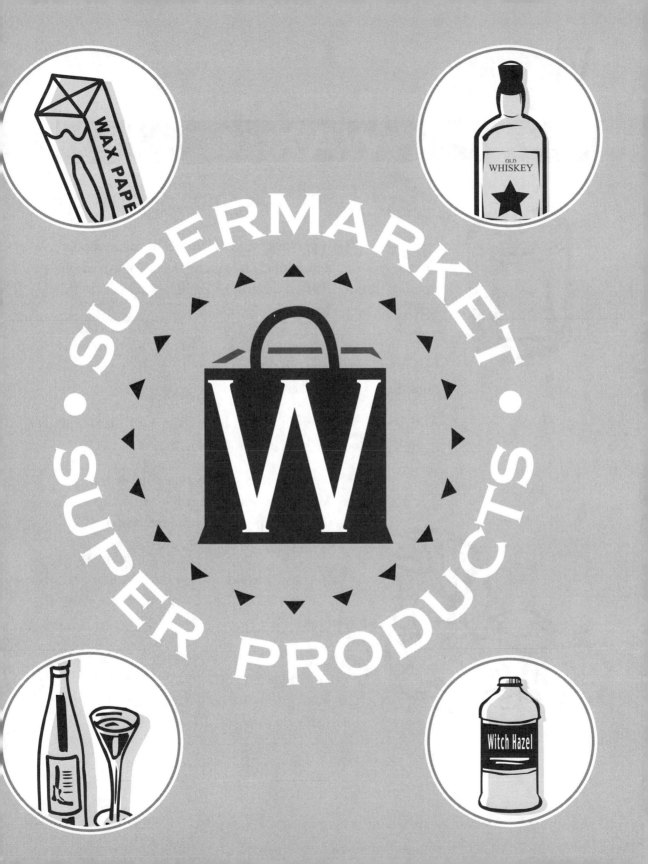

# W

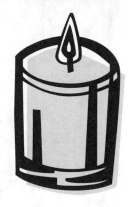

# WAX

## Home Cleaning & Upkeep

◆ To prevent chairs from scratching wooden floors, give the bottom of each leg a light coat of wax about once a month. Either paraffin or candle wax will do the trick and keep chairs gliding smoothly.

◆ Keep windows and sliding doors moving freely and quietly by rubbing wax over the gliders every now and then. It works like a charm!

◆ Use a bit of wax to keep zippers clean and running smoothly. Just rub some along the teeth.

◆ Here's an easy way to make pantyhose last longer: After every washing, rub wax on the heels and toes to keep holes from developing.

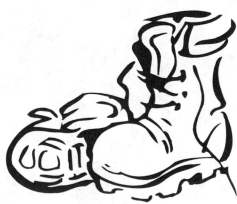

◆ When the plastic tip comes off of a shoelace, dip the end of the cord in melted wax, twist it, and let it dry. Presto—no more annoying, frayed tips!

◆ Need to reseal an envelope that you've opened, but you're out of tape *and* glue? Use wax instead. Just light a candle, and dribble the melting wax along the edge of the flap.

◆ When you're wrapping a package and run out of tape, or would rather not spoil the look with tape, just grab a candle, drip the wax between the layers of paper, and press.

◆ Do you need a new pincushion? Keep a fat candle or a chunk of paraffin close to your sewing machine to hold your needles and pins. The wax will lubricate the needles, so they'll slip through fabric more easily. (If you want something fancier than plain old wax, wrap a piece of fabric around it, or put it in a shallow, decorative dish.)

◆ Are you going camping, or headed for a summer cabin where the weather is damp? Make sure you take waterproof matches along. To make a supply of them, just light a candle, and dip each match head into the melted candle wax. Let the matches dry completely before storing them in a waterproof container.

◆ When your insulated foam cooler gets dinged, don't toss it in the trash. Instead, fill the hole with melted wax. Just be sure the wax is completely hardened before you use the cooler again.

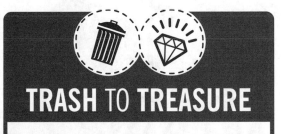

## TRASH TO TREASURE

IF YOU make homemade jellies and jams—or buy them at farmers' markets—hang on to those wax tops! Store them in an old coffee can or other covered tin, and when you've got enough, make candles. They'll smell just like the jam that was under the paraffin liner!

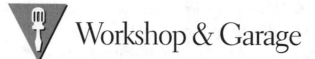

## Workshop & Garage

▼ Make your wood screws all but glide to their destination by rubbing the threads across wax before you start screwing them into the wood. (Paraffin, candle wax, and beeswax will all do the trick.)

▼ Before you paint window frames, run a candle or a chunk of paraffin all around the edge of the glass. That way, paint splatters will be a cinch to clean off.

## Yard & Garden

● After you write I.D. labels for your plants, rub a candle or a chunk of paraffin over the lettering to protect it from rain, sleet, and who-knows-what-all.

● Do you need to dig in hard soil? Put a light coat of wax on your shovel blade to help it cut through that earthy crust.

# WAX PAPER

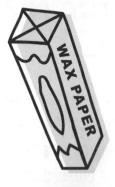

## 🏠 Home Cleaning & Upkeep

◆ Do ice cube trays or frozen-food containers tend to stick to the bottom of your freezer compartment? Make it a "no-stick" zone by lining it with a sheet of wax paper.

◆ Want to give a clean tile floor an instant glow? Just wrap a piece of wax paper around a mop, and scoot it over the floor.

◆ Shine kitchen counter-tops by rubbing them with a piece of balled-up wax paper.

◆ To keep freshly polished shoes from smearing onto clothes and furniture, wait until the polish has dried, and wipe off the excess with a piece of wax paper.

◆ Rub wax paper over metal closet rods to make hangers move back and forth more smoothly.

◆ Clean the sole plate of your iron by wiping it with wax paper. Afterwards, heat the iron slightly, and use a soft cloth to remove any excess wax.

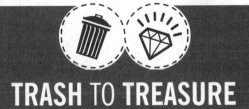

## TRASH TO TREASURE

**HERE'S A trick that will turn three kinds of trash into treasure that's hot: fire-starter nuggets for your grill or fire-place. First, cut a paper egg carton apart into 12 sections, and fill each one with either sawdust or dryer lint (only use lint that came from 100% cotton fabric). Melt down old candle nubbins or paraffin sealers from home-made jelly, and pour a layer of wax on top of the sawdust. When you want to burn, baby, burn, set one of your nuggets in the charcoal or kindling, and hold a match to the paper edge.**

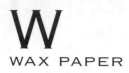

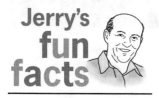

## Jerry's fun facts

Have you ever wondered how they make wax paper? A triple coating of paraffin wax is pressed onto tissue paper. The wax fills up the pores and spreads across the surface of the paper, giving it both strength and moisture resistance. And, in case you're wondering who history credits with thinking up this dandy process, it was none other than good ol' Thomas Edison!

◆ Here's a trick for keeping trousers neat-looking longer: Fold a sheet of wax paper over the leg, and iron on top of the paper. A little bit of wax will stay in the fabric, which will make the crease hold better.

◆ If you like to hand-paint clothes or other fabric items, this tip's for you: Cover your backing board with wax paper *before* you put your cloth over it. The paper will keep the paint from soaking through and making a sticky mess of the board *and* your project.

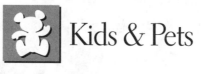

## Kids & Pets

■ When the kids are looking for a craft project, suggest this: Make sun catchers. Just shave crayons or colorful candle nubbins onto a sheet of wax paper, put another sheet of wax paper on top, and put the "sandwich" between two sheets of cloth or brown paper. Press with a low-heat iron to melt the shavings. Carefully peel off the cloth or wax paper. Let the wax cool, cut it into a fun shape, poke a hole, and hang it with a ribbon.

■ Another fun project for kids (or grownups) is to make bookmarks, placemats, and book covers. Start with leaves, flowers, or pictures from magazines. Arrange them on one piece of wax paper and cover with another piece. Then put this "sandwich" between two sheets of cloth or brown paper. Press with a low-heat iron to melt the wax in the paper and create a seal. Peel off the cloth, let cool, and cut to size (use pinking shears for a decorative edge).

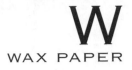

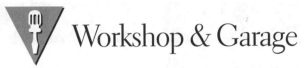

## Workshop & Garage

▼ Getting ready to put wood clamps on some freshly glued furniture? Wrap wax paper around the joints first to keep the clamps from marring the surface.

▼ For a slightly different look, use wax paper in place of a sponge for sponge-painting walls or furniture. Just scrunch it up into a ball, dip it in the paint, and dab it onto your future masterpiece!

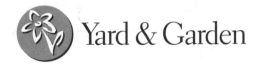

## Yard & Garden

● Tired of winding up with grass-stained trousers every time you tend your garden? Fold wax paper into squares that are three or four layers thick, and use them as kneeling pads. Or, if you're working with a small bed, run a triple-thick strip of wax paper along the entire length of the bed. The result: A tidy garden *and* clean pants!

● You need to pour a garden tonic from a bucket into a bottle, and you can't find your funnel. Don't panic—and don't spill the stuff all over the floor! Instead, lay a sheet of wax paper over a sheet of newspaper and roll it all up to form a cone, with the wax paper on the inside. Put the tip of the cone into the bottle, and pour away!

# W

# WHISKEY & RUM

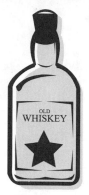

OLD WHISKEY

## ✚ Health & Beauty

 When you feel the flu coming on, this ancient remedy is still hard to beat: Boil a whole, large, tart, juicy apple in a quart of water until the apple falls apart. Strain out the solids, and add a cup of whiskey and about ½ teaspoon of lemon juice. Sweeten to taste with honey if you like. Then get into bed and drink the toddy. If you've acted in time, by morning, those germs will be history! If you'd like a slightly milder cure, add a shot of whiskey and a little honey to a mug of warm milk, and drift off to dreamland.

 When you cut yourself and there's no antiseptic around, reach for the whiskey, and pour some on. It's not the cheapest way to clean a wound and kill bacteria, but it sure works!

 Are you suffering from arthritis or rheumatism? Folks I know swear by this cure: Steep 3 tablespoons of sassafras root in a fifth of whiskey for 24 hours. Take 1 tablespoon three times a day before meals. (You'll find sassafras root in health-food stores and in the health-food section of many large supermarkets.)

 Lighten freckles and sun spots by dabbing the marks several times a day with a mixture of 1 tablespoon of light rum, 2 tablespoons of fresh lemon juice, and 1 teaspoon of glycerin. Store the mixture in a glass bottle with a tight lid.

# Yard & Garden

● Keep your herbs happy and healthy by feeding them every six weeks with a solution of 1 cup of tea and ½ tablespoon each of bourbon (or other whiskey), ammonia, and hydrogen peroxide mixed in 1 gallon of warm water.

● After you root-prune any shrub, pour ¼ pound of Epsom salts evenly into the cuts, all the way around the plant. Then pour this elixir over the Epsom salts: 1 can of beer, 4 tablespoons of instant tea granules, and 1 tablespoon each of whiskey, baby shampoo, ammonia, and hydrogen peroxide mixed in 2 gallons of very warm water.

● To get direct-sown flower or vegetable seeds off to a rip-roaring start, spray the soil daily with a solution of 1 teaspoon each of whiskey, ammonia, and dishwashing liquid per quart of weak tea in a hand-held spray bottle.

### REMARKABLE RECIPES

## ALL-FACES MASQUE

Here's a masque that works for any skin type—simply by altering one ingredient.

**1 egg***
**Juice of 1 lemon**
**¼ cup of nonfat powdered milk**
**1 tbsp. of whiskey**

Mix all of the ingredients together. Smooth the mixture over your face, avoiding the eye area. Let it dry, and remove it with a warm, wet washcloth. Keep the mixture in a jar in the refrigerator, and use it once a week.

*\* For normal skin, use the whole egg; for dry skin, use only the yolk; for oily skin, use only the white.*

● When winter has finally passed, help your shrubs spring into action by watering them with a mixture of 4 tablespoons each of bourbon (or other whiskey) and instant tea granules and 2 tablespoons of dishwashing liquid in 2 gallons of warm water.

● Keep potted perennials happy with this tonic: Mix 2 tablespoons of rum, 1 tablespoon of all-purpose (15-30-15) fertilizer, ½ teaspoon of unflavored gelatin, and ¼ teaspoon of instant tea granules in a 1-gallon jug. Fill the jug with water. When watering time rolls around, add ½ cup of this mix per gallon of water.

● Your houseplants will have the healthiest, lushest foliage in town if you feed them with this mix: ½ tablespoon each of bourbon (or other whiskey), ammonia, and hydrogen peroxide; ¼ teaspoon of instant tea granules; and 1 multivitamin tablet with iron mixed in 1 gallon of warm water.

**REMARKABLE RECIPES**

## TRANSPLANT TONIC

For a tree or shrub, being transplanted is a shocking experience. This soothing drink will ease the stress of going from a nursery pot, or the bare-root wrappings, to the wide-open spaces of your yard.

⅓ **cup of hydrogen peroxide**
¼ **cup of whiskey**
¼ **cup of instant tea granules**
¼ **cup of baby shampoo**
2 **tbsp. of Fish Emulsion (a fertilizer that's available at garden centers)**
1 **gal. of water**

Mix all of these ingredients in a big bucket, and pour the solution into the new planting hole.

# WINE

 ## Health & Beauty

🍎 Control acne breakouts by dabbing a little wine on the zits. Use white wine for fair skin, red for darker complexions.

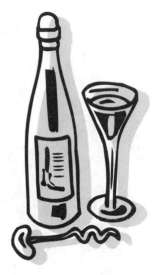

🍎 Want to add golden highlights to your hair? Try this time-honored trick: Heat 2 cups of white wine (don't boil it!), add 3 tablespoons of chopped rhubarb stems, remove it from the stove, and let it steep for 10 minutes. Shampoo as usual, rinse with the potion, and partially dry your hair with a towel. Then sit in the sun to finish the job. Repeat the process until your tresses reach the desired shade of pale. Be sure to give your hair a good rinse with clear, warm water.

🍎 Has swimming in a chlorinated pool given your blonde hair a greenish tinge? Pour yourself a glass of red wine—don't drink it, though! Instead, pour it on your head. Work it through the strands, follow up with your normal shampoo, and that'll be the end of the green-hair blues!

Here's a simple skin freshener that your face will love: Put 1 cup of white wine and 1 sliced lemon in a glass or enamel pot, and bring it to a boil over medium heat (or put it in a microwave-safe bowl and bring to a boil—about 1½ minutes on high). Boil it for another full minute, remove the pan from the heat, and stir in 1 tablespoon of sugar. Let the mixture cool, strain it, and store it in a tightly capped bottle. Whenever you feel the need for facial refreshment, just dab the lotion onto your skin with a cotton ball.

Use white wine to relieve sunburn. Just spritz the wine directly onto the stricken skin, and don't rub! When the liquid has evaporated, apply a moisturizing lotion.

Cut yourself? Pour some wine onto the wound. Chemicals called *polyphenols* in the wine will kill bacteria and prevent infection.

Do you have a cough that's keeping you awake at night? Here's what to do: Heat a cup of red wine (don't let it boil!), and add lemon, cinnamon, and sugar to taste. You'll sleep like a baby!

## REMARKABLE RECIPES

## WINE & APPLE MASQUE

Here's a recipe that will slough off dead skin cells, refine your pores, and gradually even out your skin tone.

**2 tbsp. of ground oatmeal***
**2 tsp. of red wine**
**2 tsp. of apple juice**

Mix the oatmeal, wine, and apple juice in small bowl until it forms a spreadable paste (add more liquid if you need to). Smooth the mixture onto your face and neck, and leave it on for 20 to 30 minutes, until dry. Rinse your face with warm water and pat dry.

*\* Grind the oatmeal to a powder in a blender or coffee grinder.*

## ⌂ Home Cleaning & Upkeep

◆ Are cockroaches invading your kitchen? Buy the cheapest wine you can find, pour it into saucers, and set them around the room. The roaches will throng to the party, lift their glasses (so to speak), and die happy!

◆ When you want a really no-muss, no-fuss egg dye, use plain red wine. It will color the shells a pretty shade of purple. Just put hard-boiled eggs in a bowl, pour in enough wine to cover them, put them in the refrigerator, and let them sit until they reach the color you desire.

◆ Get sticky residue off glass, ceramic, or Formica® by rubbing with a sponge that's been dipped in white wine. The alcohol will dissolve the sticky stuff. Follow this up with a cool-water wipedown.

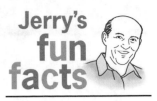

**Jerry's fun facts**

The American wine-making industry owes its start to a Franciscan missionary from Spain, Padre Junípero Serra. He picked up some grapevines on his journey through Mexico and planted them when he arrived in San Diego in 1769. A few years later, the country's first winery was built nearby. The Franciscan fathers took grapes with them when they ventured north to found the Sonoma Mission in 1823. And the rest, as they say, is history!

# W

# WITCH HAZEL

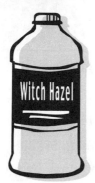

## ✚ Health & Beauty

❧ Make a healthful skin toner by mixing 1 teaspoon of green tea leaves in ½ cup of witch hazel. Gently dab the mixture onto your face and neck with a cotton pad. There's no need to rinse.

❧ Here's a triple-threat tonic that tightens pores, soothes sunburn and other minor burns, and even works as a gentle deodorant: Mix 1 cup of witch hazel, 3 tablespoons of coarsely chopped cucumber, and the juice of 1 lemon in a clean, glass jar with a lid. Let it sit for two days, strain out the cucumber, and pour the liquid into a bottle. Keep it in the refrigerator, and dab it on with a cotton ball whenever the need arises.

❧ To ease sunburn pain fast, dip gauze or cheesecloth in witch hazel, and gently wrap it around the affected area. As the cloth dries, repeat the procedure until you feel relief. Follow up with a rich moisturizing lotion. If the sun has done its number on a part of your body that's not easily wrappable, you've got two other great cooling options: Either pour some witch hazel into a spray bottle and spritz your sore skin, or soak in a tepid bath with 1 to 2 cups of witch hazel added to the water.

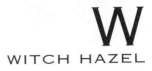

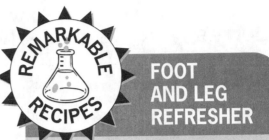

🍎 You were standing in the wrong place when the wind caught the door, and you wound up with a shiner the size of a dinner plate. Now what do you do? Just soak a wash cloth in witch hazel, and hold it over your eye. The pain and swelling will vamoose. Make sure you don't get any *in* your eye, though, because it will sting like crazy!

🍎 Are hemorrhoids making your life miserable? Reduce the swelling and relieve the burn and itching with witch hazel—the active ingredient in over-the-counter hemorrhoid treatments. Keep the bottle in the refrigerator, then drizzle some on a sterile gauze pad, and hold it against the sore spots. Repeat the procedure three or four times a day, or as often as you feel the need.

🍎 Stop the itch of poison ivy and insect bites by making a paste of witch hazel and baking soda. Smooth it onto the rash for fast relief.

🍎 When the weather turns steamy, keep your cool by misting your skin with this elixir: Mix 2 teaspoons of witch hazel, 10 drops of peppermint essential oil, and 12 drops of lavender essential oil in an 8-ounce spray bottle, filling the balance of the bottle with water. Keep it in the refrigerator, and reach for it anytime you feel too darn hot.

## FOOT AND LEG REFRESHER

When you do more walking than you're used to, or you've been standing up all day long, give your legs and feet a refreshing treat with this gel.

**½ cup of aloe vera gel**
**1 tbsp. of witch hazel**
**1½ tsp. of cornstarch**
**3–4 drops of peppermint extract**

Mix the aloe vera, witch hazel, and cornstarch in a microwave-safe container. Nuke it on high for 1 to 2 minutes, stirring every 30 seconds, until the mixture is about the consistency of honey. Let it cool, stir in the peppermint extract, and store the gel in an airtight container. Smooth it on your tired, aching feet and legs, wait 10 to 15 minutes, and rinse with warm water. You'll feel like running a marathon! (Well, almost.)

# W

## WITCH HAZEL

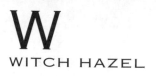
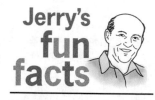
No one knows for sure how witch hazel (*Hamamelis virginiana*) got its name, but it has nothing to do with witches or witchcraft. Our Pilgrim fathers used the shrub's forked branches to dowse for underground water. In those days, the word *wych* meant small and lively, which described the dowsing rod as it bobbed up and down in the diviner's hands. Over the years, *wych* evolved into *witch*. As for who Hazel was, your guess is as good as mine!

 Want a *really* simple alternative to commercial aftershaves? Just mix 1 part witch hazel and 1 part apple cider vinegar, and slap it on your face. It's refreshing!

 If your skin is extra-oily, keep plenty of witch hazel on hand. It's the perfect balancing agent. Just dab it on your face with a clean cotton ball in the morning and before bed—or whenever you get that oily feeling.

 Make a spray deodorant by mixing ½ cup of witch hazel with 2 tablespoons of vodka, 1 tablespoon of glycerin, and ½ teaspoon of Liquid Chlorophyll (see the recipe on page 316). Pour the solution into a hand-held spray bottle, and spritz your underarms morning, noon, and/or night.

 Hey, guys! Is your skin too sensitive for regular aftershave lotions? Use this extra-gentle formula instead: Just mix ½ cup of witch hazel with 2 tablespoons each of vodka and dried chamomile flowers in a clean jar with a tight-fitting lid. Let it steep in a cool, dark place for two weeks, strain out the solids, and splash it on.

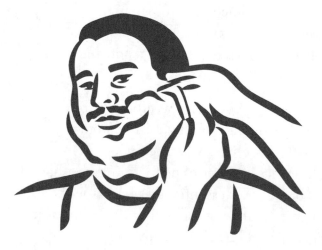

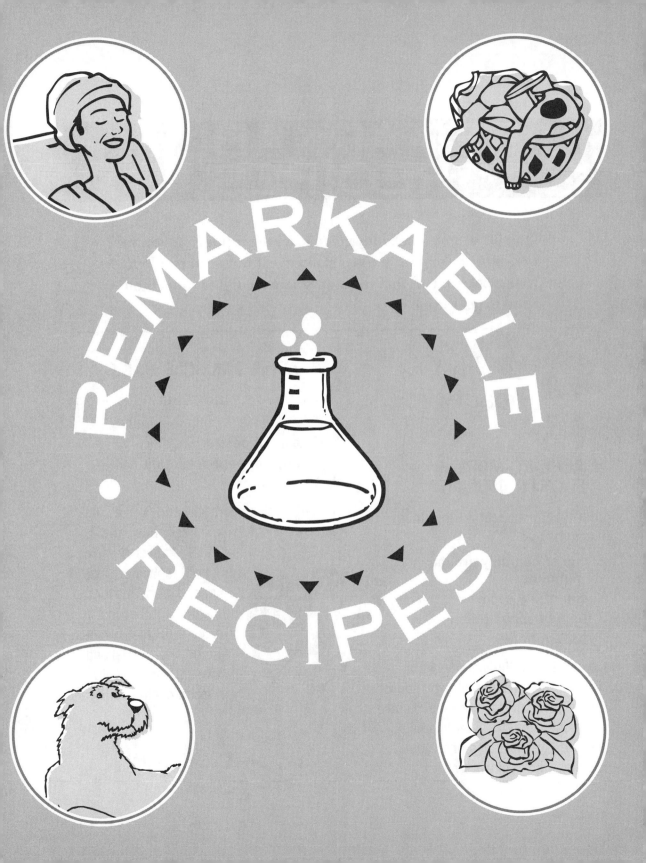

# REMARKABLE RECIPES

Use this section as a handy guide to all the recipes and tonics in this book. You can see at a glance what you need to add to your grocery list, so that you always have the right products on hand to get the job done!

## Health & Beauty

### ACHE-NO-MORE FOOT FORMULA

Your tired, achy feet will love this nighttime treat.

¼ cup of coarsely ground almonds
¼ cup of dry oatmeal
3 tbsp. of cocoa butter
2 tbsp. of honey

Combine all of the ingredients, and massage the mixture into your skin. Pull on clean cotton socks, and leave them on overnight. In the morning, remove the socks and rinse your tootsies with cool water.

### ACHING MUSCLE MAGIC

Ease aching muscles with a little of this minty remedy.

1 tbsp. of petroleum jelly
6 drops of peppermint oil
Warm water

Mix the petroleum jelly and oil in a small bowl, and put it in a larger bowl of warm water. Soak a towel in warm (not hot!) tap water, wring it out, and drape it over the trouble spot. Leave it in place for 3 to 4 minutes. Remove the towel and massage the oil/jelly mixture into your skin.

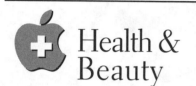

## ❤ AHHH AFTERSHAVE

Okay, guys—this one's for you. Here's an easy recipe that will make the women in your life go "Ahhh."

**2 cups of rubbing alcohol**
**1 tbsp. of glycerin**
**1 tbsp. of dried lavender**
**1 tsp. of dried rosemary**
**1 tsp. of ground cloves**

Mix all of the ingredients well, pour into a bottle with a tight-fitting cap, and refrigerate. Shake well before using, and strain as you use it. This aftershave will keep, refrigerated, for up to two months.

## ❤ ALL EYES ARE ON YOU

Here's a great recipe for a gentle and soothing eye-makeup remover.

**1 tbsp. of castor oil**
**1 tbsp. of olive oil**
**2 tsp. of canola oil**

Mix all of the ingredients together. Apply with a tissue or cotton ball to remove eye shadow, eyeliner, or mascara safely and without irritation. Discard any of the remaining oil mixture.

## ❤ ALL-FACES MASQUE

Here's a masque that works for any skin type—simply by altering one ingredient.

**1 egg***
**Juice of 1 lemon**
**¼ cup of nonfat powdered milk**
**1 tbsp. of whiskey**

Mix all of the ingredients together. Smooth the mixture over your face, avoiding the eye area. Let it dry, and remove it with a warm, wet washcloth. Keep the mixture in the refrigerator, and use it once a week.

*For normal skin, use the whole egg; for dry skin, use only the yolk; for oily skin, use only the white.*

## ALMOND FACE CLEANSER

Here's a facial cleanser that's perfect for all skin types, and you can put it together in a flash.

**1 cup of shelled almonds**
**1 cup of dry oatmeal**
**1 cup of dried orange peel**

Put all of the ingredients in a blender or food processor, and chop until they form a fine powder. Scoop some into the palm of your hand, add a few drops of water, and rub it onto your face. (Be careful not to get any in your eyes.) Rinse with warm water, and pat dry. Store the powder in an airtight container at room temperature.

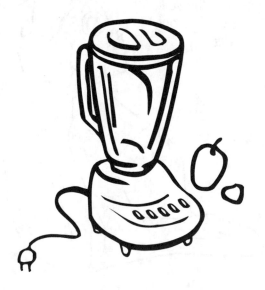

## ANTI-AGE LOTION

If age and too much time in the sun have left you with spotty skin, lighten those splotches with this tonic.

**Juice of 1 lime**
**Juice of 1 lemon**
**4 tbsp. of plain yogurt**
**2 tbsp. of honey**

Mix all of the ingredients together, and gently massage the lotion into each spot at least once a week. Store the mixture in a covered container in the refrigerator.

## APPLE ASTRINGENT

The acids in apple juice tone your skin and help keep it clear—and they're mild enough for even sensitive skin.

**½ cup of apple juice**
**4 tbsp. of vodka (100 proof)**
**1 tbsp. of honey**
**1 tsp. of sea salt**

Pour all of the ingredients into a bottle with a tight cap and shake well. Apply the solution to your face and neck twice a day with a cotton pad.

## APPLE-OATMEAL FACIAL

Here's a simple formula that will slough off dead skin cells, refine pores, and even out your skin tone.

**1 tbsp. of ground oatmeal***
**2 tsp. of apple juice**
**2 tsp. of red wine**
**1 tsp. of honey**

In a small bowl, mix the oatmeal with the apple juice, wine, and honey to make a paste. (Add more liquid if you need to.) Spread the mixture onto your face and throat, let it dry for 30 minutes, and rinse with warm water.

*\* Grind the dry oatmeal in a blender or coffee grinder.*

## BACK-IN-BALANCE BATH

Muscle aches, spasms, and cramps could be a signal that your internal electrolytes are out of balance. To make things right, reach for this recipe.

**2 cups of Epsom salts**
**2 cups of kosher or
    sea salt**
**2 tbsp. of potassium
    crystals***

Pour the salts and crystals into a tub of hot water, and soak your aches and pains away.

*\* Available in the health-food section of large supermarkets, and in most health-food stores.*

## BATH SALTS, OVER EASY

Luxury bath treats don't come any easier than this formula!

**1 cup of Epsom salts**
**1 cup of table salt**
**1 cup of baking soda**

Combine the salts and soda, and store the mixture in an airtight container at room temperature. At bath time, pour about 2 tablespoons into running water. For an aromatic bath, add a few drops of your favorite essential oil as the tub fills.

## 🍎 BAY RUM AFTERSHAVE

If you're looking for a homemade gift idea for the men in your life, this classic potion is the perfect answer.

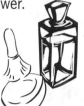

½ cup of vodka
2 tbsp. of dark rum
2 dried bay leaves
¼ tsp. of allspice
1 cinnamon stick
Rind from 1 small orange, shredded

Mix all of the ingredients together. Pour the mixture into a clean jar with a tight lid, and set it in a cool, dark place for two weeks. Strain out the solids, and pour the liquid into a nice-looking bottle.

## 🍎 BERRY GOOD FACIAL MASQUE

When your skin is craving nourishment and moisture, this masque's the berries!

3–4 ripe, medium-sized strawberries
1 tbsp. of evaporated milk
1 tbsp. of honey
1 tsp. of cornstarch (optional)

Purée the berries in a blender or food processor. In a bowl, mix the purée with the milk and honey. If it's too runny, add the cornstarch. Apply to your face and neck, leave on for 10 minutes, and rinse.

## 🍎 BLACKHEADS-BE-GONE FACIAL PASTE

Banish blackheads with this simple, but effective formula.

1 egg white
1 part dry oatmeal
1 part honey

Mix the ingredients together to make a paste, adding more oatmeal or honey as necessary. Smooth the mixture onto your face, and wait 10 minutes or so. Rinse with warm water, and pat dry.

## 🍎 BRING ON THE BUBBLES!

If your idea of relaxation is sinking into a tub full of bubbles, this recipe's for you!

1 gal. of water
2 cups of soap flakes
½ cup of glycerin
2 cups of shampoo
Scented oil (optional)

Mix the water, soap, and 2 tablespoons of the glycerin in a pot over low heat, stirring until the soap flakes have dissolved. In a large bowl, add this mixture to the rest of the glycerin, the shampoo and, if you'd like, scented oil. Store in quart containers at room temperature. To use, add 1 cup to the water as your tub is filling.

## CHOCOLATE LIP BALM

When harsh winter air leaves your lips cracked and dry, reach for this recipe. While you're at it, make a few extras as gifts for all the choc-aholics in your life!

**2 tbsp. of petroleum jelly**
**1 tbsp. of powdered chocolate milk mix (or to taste)***
**1 vitamin E capsule**

Put the petroleum jelly into a microwave-safe container, and nuke it at 30-second intervals until the jelly is melted. (Be patient—it might take several minutes.) Snip open the capsule and pour the vitamin E oil into the melted petroleum jelly, and then stir. Mix in the chocolate milk powder, return it to the microwave for another 30 seconds, and mix again until smooth. Let the mixture cool, and pour it into small, clean, airtight containers.

*Or use vanilla or strawberry milk mix.*

## CITRUS-SPICY MOUTHWASH

Looking for a new brand of mouthwash? Try this simple, spicy solution.

**¼ cup of vodka**
**¼ cup of water**
**5 drops of cinnamon oil**
**5 drops of clove oil**
**5 drops of orange oil**

Combine all of the ingredients, and store the mixture in a dark-colored glass bottle with a spray top. Shake well before using.

## CLEAN-AND-SOFT FACIAL SCRUB

For skin that's squeaky clean *and* as soft as silk, reach for this remarkable recipe.

**2 tbsp. of ground almonds***
**2 tsp. of milk**
**½ tsp. of flour**
**½ tsp. of honey**

Mix the almond powder with the milk, flour, and honey to make a thick paste. (If it's too thick or too thin, add more milk or flour as necessary.) Rub the mixture into your skin, and rinse with warm water.

*Grind the almonds to a fine powder in a blender or coffee grinder.*

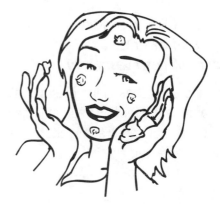

## COMB-AND-BRUSH CLEANER

Here's a simple formula for getting your hairbrushes and combs sparkling clean.

**¼ cup of dishwashing liquid**
**¼ cup of ammonia**
**2 cups of water**

Mix all of these ingredients together, and soak your combs and brushes in the solution for 5 to 10 minutes. Remove them, and scrape the brushes with the combs, and vice versa. Rinse with cool water, and let them dry.

## CREAM DEODORANT

This simple concoction will keep you feeling as fresh and dry as any store-bought brand.

**2 tbsp. of baby powder**
**2 tbsp. of baking soda**
**2 tbsp. of petroleum jelly**

Combine all of these ingredients in a pan, and heat over low heat until the mixture is smooth and creamy. Store it in an airtight container.

## DEEP-CLEANING FACIAL FORMULA

Get your skin deep-down clean—and satiny soft—with this easy masque.

**½ of an avocado**
**2 tbsp. of orange juice**
**1 tsp. of molasses**
**1 tsp. of honey**

Mix all of the ingredients in a blender or food processor. Smooth the mixture onto your skin, wait 30 to 40 minutes, and remove the masque using a damp, warm washcloth. Store extra formula in a covered container in the refrigerator; it will keep for two or three days.

## EASY CALLUS REMOVER

This formula will gently remove those annoying calluses that develop in the palms of your hands from canes or tools.

**1–2 tbsp. of cornmeal**
**1 tbsp. of avocado oil**

Mix the ingredients to form a paste with a meal-like texture. Take the mixture in the palm of your hand, and rub both hands together, working the gritty stuff into the calluses and around your fingers. Repeat once or twice a week.

## ❦ EASY ENERGIZING BATH

When hot, muggy weather lays you flat (or anytime you need a quick pick-me-up), pour this formula into your bathtub.

**½ cup of lime juice**
**½ cup of lemon juice**
**5–6 drops of lemon extract**
**½ cup of baking soda\***

Mix all of the ingredients in a bowl, pour the solution into tepid bathwater, and ease into the tub. When you get out, you'll be ready for action!

*\*Add soda only if you have hard water.*

## ❦ EASY, FANCY BATH SALTS

If you prefer scent *and* color in your bathwater, this is the recipe for you.

**1 cup of Epsom salts**
**4 drops of food coloring**
**4 drops of scented oil**

Pour the Epsom salts, food coloring, and your favorite scented oil into a zipper-lock plastic bag. Shake and knead it to blend the color and scent, and pour the mixture into an airtight jar. At bath time, pour ½ cup into running water, sink in, and luxuriate!

## ❦ EASY HERBAL VINEGAR

Just about anything that plain vinegar can do, herbal vinegar can do better! Besides adding pizzazz to any recipe, it's like a combination first-aid kit and beauty spa in a bottle. And, it couldn't be easier to make!

**½ cup of dried herbs, or 1 cup of fresh herb leaves (washed and dried)**
**2 cups of white vinegar**

Put the herbs in a sterilized glass jar, and mash them slightly with a spoon. Pour the vinegar over the herbs, cover the jar tightly, and let the mixture steep in a dark place at room temperature for one to three weeks. Shake the jar every few days, and taste the vinegar once a week until the flavor reaches the desired intensity. Add more herbs if you need to. When the flavor suits you, strain out the solids, and pour the vinegar into a sterilized bottle with a tight cap. Keep it away from direct light, which rapidly decreases the herbs' potency.

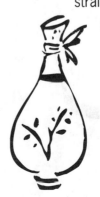

## 🍎 ENERGIZING ELIXIR

Long before sports drinks came on the market, folks took a break from hard work or play by sitting under a shady tree and drinking this restorative beverage.

**2 ½ cups of sugar**
**1 cup of dark molasses**
**½ cup of vinegar (either white or cider)**
**1 gal. of water**

Mix all of the ingredients together in a big jug. Then get your team out of the sun, and pour everyone a nice, tall refreshing glass.

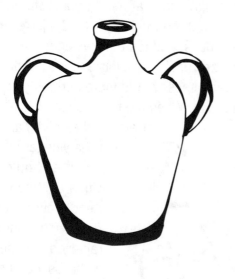

## 🍎 FABULOUS FRECKLE FADER

Lighten sun spots and freckles with this marvelous mixture.

**2 tbsp. of fresh lemon juice**
**1 tbsp. of light rum**
**1 tsp. of glycerin**

Combine all of the ingredients in a glass bottle with a tight lid, and shake to blend. Several times a day, dab the mixture onto your spots with a cotton ball. Before you know it, the marks will be ghosts of their former selves.

## 🍎 FACE FOOD

You'd be hard-pressed to find a more skin-pleasing fruit than an avocado. Its high fat content makes it the perfect base for a nourishing masque.

**½ of an avocado**
**1 tbsp. of plain yogurt**
**½ tsp. of vitamin E oil**

Mash the avocado, then blend in the yogurt and vitamin E oil. Smooth the mixture onto your face, paying close attention to the fine lines around your eyes and mouth. Leave the masque on for about 20 minutes, and rinse with warm water.

## 🍎 FACIAL POWER MASQUE

When your skin needs powerful, but gentle, scrubbing action, use this heavy-duty cleanser/masque.

**½ cup of dry oatmeal**
**1 tbsp. of honey**
**1 tbsp. of cider vinegar**
**1 tsp. of ground almonds**

Mix all of the ingredients in a bowl. Moisten your face with a warm wash-cloth. With your hands, smooth the mixture onto your skin, avoiding the eye area. Wait until the masque dries, and remove it with a warm, damp washcloth.

## 🍎 FLEE, FLU FORMULA

Before cold and flu season starts, arm yourself with this tonic.

**¾ cup of vodka**
**2½ tbsp. of dried echinacea root***
**¾ cup of distilled water**

Mix the ingredients in a glass jar with a tight lid. Store in a cool, dark place for two weeks, and strain into glass bottles. At the first sign of cold or flu, mix 2 or 3 drops in a glass of water, and drink up!

*Available in the health-food section of large supermarkets, and in most health-food stores.*

## 🍎 FOAMING BATH CRYSTALS

When you need to soothe frayed nerves or relax aching muscles, it's good to have a jar of these colorful crystals on hand. (They make great gifts, too.)

**6 cups of rock salt**
**½ cup of mild dishwashing liquid**
**1 tbsp. of vegetable oil**
**4–5 drops of food coloring**

Put the rock salt in a bowl. In another bowl, mix the dishwashing liquid, vegetable oil, and food coloring together, and pour the solution over the salt. Stir to coat the crystals, and spread them out on wax paper. When they're completely dry (usually in about 24 hours), put them in a jar. At bath time, pour ¼ cup of the crystals into the tub under running water.

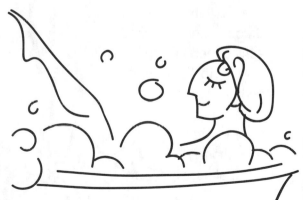

# FOOT AND LEG REFRESHER

When you do more walking than you're used to, or you're standing all day, or you spent last night "cutting a rug," give your legs and feet a refreshing treat with this gel.

**½ cup of aloe vera gel**
**1 tbsp. of witch hazel**
**1½ tsp. of cornstarch**
**3–4 drops of peppermint extract**

Mix the aloe vera, witch hazel, and cornstarch in a microwave-safe container. Nuke it on high for 1 to 2 minutes, stirring every 30 seconds, until the mixture is about the consistency of honey. Let it cool, stir in the peppermint extract, and store the gel in an airtight container. Smooth it on your tired, aching feet and legs, wait 10 to 15 minutes, and rinse with warm water. You'll feel like running a marathon! (Well, almost.)

# FOOT SOOTHER & SMOOTHER

Say goodbye to rough, cracked skin on your feet with this soothing solution.

**1 tbsp. of almond oil**
**1 tbsp. of olive oil**
**1 tsp. of wheat germ**

Combine all of the ingredients, and store the mixture in a bottle with a tight cap. Shake well before using. Rub generously into feet and heels, especially the dry parts. Your tootsies will love you for it!

# FRAGRANT BATH CRYSTALS

Mix up a batch of this beautiful blend, and soak your troubles away. While you're at it, make a few more batches to give as presents.

**½ cup of Epsom salts**
**½ cup of sea salt**
**½ cup of fresh lavender, chamomile, or rose buds**
**¼ cup of baking soda**
**15 drops of fragrance oil (any kind you like to match or complement the flowers' fragrance)**
**Food coloring (optional)**

Blend the salts, flowers, and baking soda in a blender or food processor.

Let the mixture sit for 30 minutes or so to dry a little, then add the oil and food coloring. Pour the blend into jars.

## FRUITY FIX-UP

If your hair is dry, frizzy, or damaged, this healthful concoction will set it right, fast!

½ of a ripe banana
½ of a ripe avocado
1 tbsp. of extra-virgin olive oil
3 drops of lemon oil

Mash the banana and avocado together in a bowl, then mix in the olive oil and lemon oil. Work the mixture into your hair

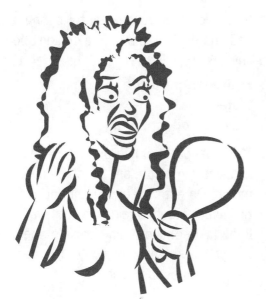

(don't wet your hair first), and cover it with a shower cap. Wait about 60 minutes, and shampoo as usual. For badly damaged hair, repeat this treatment up to three times a week until the bounce and shine return.

## FRUITY FOOT REVIVER

Been on your feet all day? Revive those tired dogs with this fruity treat.

8 strawberries, mashed
2 tbsp. of olive oil
1 tsp. of sea salt or kosher salt

Mix the ingredients together to form a paste. Massage it into your feet, rinse it off, and dry with a soft towel.

## GET-A-MOVE-ON MIX

When constipation strikes, ease the discomfort with this classic remedy.

½ cup of applesauce
4–6 prunes, chopped
1 tbsp. of bran

Mix all of the ingredients together, and eat the concoction just before you go to bed. By morning, things should be on the move again!

## ❖ HAIR-TAMING TREATMENT

When your hair is so dry it's about to split, bring those ends under control with this sweet and pungent tamer.

**2 tbsp. of garlic oil**
**1 tsp. of honey**
**1 egg yolk**

Combine the oil and honey, then beat in the egg yolk. Rub the mixture into your hair a small section at a time. Cover your hair with a shower cap or a plastic bag, and wait 30 minutes. Rinse thoroughly, and shampoo as usual.

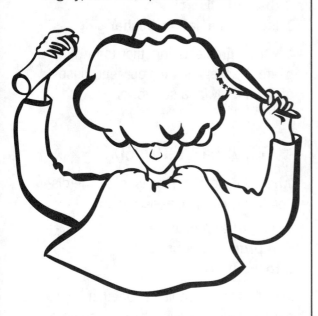

## ❖ HAIR'S-TO-BANANAS HAIR CREAM

Revive dry or damaged hair with this creamy concoction.

**1 banana**
**1 tbsp. of mayonnaise**
**1 tbsp. of olive oil**

Purée the banana in a blender until it's smooth and lump-free. Add the mayonnaise and olive oil, and blend until creamy. Massage the mixture into your hair, wait 15 to 30 minutes, rinse with warm water, and shampoo as usual.

## ❖ HALITOSIS HELPER

Good old peroxide is great for curing bad breath. And, the recipe couldn't be any easier!

**Hydrogen peroxide**
**Water**
**Flavored oil (optional)**

Mix equal parts of hydrogen peroxide and water in a cup, and swish it in your mouth. Do not swallow! Spit it out and rinse your mouth again with cool water. If the taste of hydrogen peroxide doesn't suit you, add a drop or two of flavored oil, such as peppermint.

## ☙ HEIRLOOM FLU STOPPER

When you feel the flu coming on, this ancient remedy is still hard to beat.

**1 large, tart, juicy apple**
**1 qt. of water**
**2 shots of whiskey**
**½ tsp. of lemon juice**
**Honey (optional)**

Boil the apple in the water until the apple falls apart in pieces. Strain out the solids, and add the whiskey and lemon juice. Sweeten to taste with honey, if you like. Then get into bed and drink the toddy. If you've acted in time, by morning, those germs will be history!

## ☙ HOMEMADE COLD CREAM

You *could* go out and pay a lot of money for a fancy cold cream. Or, you could make your own with this easy recipe.

**1 egg yolk**
**2 tbsp. of lemon juice**
**½ cup of light vegetable oil**
**½ cup of olive oil**

Combine the egg yolk and lemon juice, and mix with a wire whisk. Gradually add the oils, continuing to stir, until the mixture thickens. If it's too thick, add more lemon juice; if it's too thin, add a little more egg yolk. Store in a covered container in the refrigerator.

## ☙ HOMEMADE SHAMPOO

Who needs store-bought shampoo when you can make your own? Here's the simple recipe.

**¼ cup of liquid castile soap**
**½ tsp. of light vegetable oil**
**¼ cup of water**

Combine all of these ingredients, and pour the mixture into a clean, empty pump or squeeze bottle. (If your hair is very oily, omit the vegetable oil.)

## ❦ HONEY & CUCUMBER CLEANSER

When you want to soothe and revitalize your skin at the same time, whip up this simple lotion.

**¼ of a small cucumber, peeled and seeded**
**2 tbsp. of honey**
**1 tbsp. of whole milk**

Purée the cucumber, strain it, and pour its juice into a bowl. Mix in the honey, add the milk, and stir. Using cotton pads, apply the mixture to your face and neck. Wait 20 minutes, then rinse.

## ❦ HONEY OF A FACIAL

When you whip up this recipe, it will look good enough to eat—but use it to soothe and soften your face instead!

**2 egg whites**
**2 tbsp. of honey**
**2 tbsp. of mashed avocado**

Thoroughly mix all of the ingredients in a small bowl, and using your fingers, apply the mixture to your face. Leave it on for 30 minutes, rinse with warm water, and pat dry.

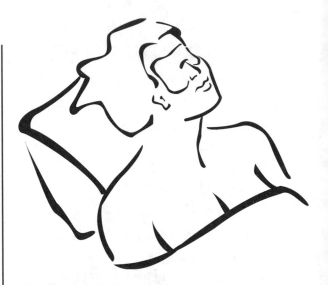

## ❦ HOW-SWEET-IT-IS MOISTURE MASQUE

Soften and nourish your skin with this sweet-smelling facial.

**2 tbsp. of mashed strawberries**
**1 tbsp. of coconut oil**
**1 tbsp. of olive oil**
**1 tbsp. of vegetable oil**
**2 drops of vitamin E oil**
**Witch hazel**

Combine the berries and oils in a bowl. Smooth the mixture sparingly onto your face and go about your business for a few hours. Then rinse with warm water, and use a cotton pad to pat your face with witch hazel. Store any leftover masque in a covered container in the refrigerator, and use within a few days.

## ● IN-FROM-THE-OUTDOORS REFRESHING FACIAL

If you've been spending more time than usual in the great outdoors, treat yourself to this rejuvenating facial.

**5 vitamin E capsules**
**2 tsp. of plain yogurt**
**½ tsp. of honey**
**½ tsp. of lemon juice**

Prick the vitamin E capsules and drain the contents into a bowl. Add the yogurt, honey, and lemon juice, and mix well. Apply the mixture to your face with a cotton ball, wait about 10 minutes, and rinse with warm water.

## ● LEMON FACE CREAM

Use this cream every night to keep your skin satiny soft.

**1 lemon**
**¼ cup or so of heavy cream (whipping cream)**
**Piece of muslin or other light cloth**

From the center of the lemon, cut a slice that's about ¼ inch thick. Lay it flat in a clean glass jar that has a lid. Pour in enough cream to cover the lemon slice, cover the container with the cloth, and let it sit at room temperature for 24 hours, or until it's about the thickness of face cream. Replace the cloth with the regular jar lid, and put it in the refrigerator. Rub the cream into your skin every night at bedtime. The mixture will eventually spoil, so make a new batch every week.

## ● LEMON-FRESH HAIR SPRAY

Tired of store-bought hair sprays? Try this super-simple alternative.

**2 cups of water**
**2 lemons**
**1 tbsp. of vodka**

Boil the water in a saucepan. While the water is boiling, peel and finely chop the lemons. Add them to the boiling water, and simmer over low heat until the lemons are soft. Cool, strain, and pour into a spray bottle. Add the vodka, and shake well. If the solution is too sticky, dilute it with a little water.

## 🍎 LIGHTEN-UP HAIR FORMULA

If you'd like to lighten you hair without chemicals—or a beauty shop price tag—this formula is just for you.

**2 tbsp. of mild shampoo**
**Juice of 2 limes**
**Juice of 1 lemon**

Mix the shampoo and juices, pour the solution onto your hair, and massage it in. Sit in the sun or under a helmet-type hair dryer for 15 to 20 minutes, then rinse thoroughly.

## 🍎 LIQUID CHLOROPHYLL

Looking for a new deodorant? Whip up a batch of this fresh-smelling brew.

**Grass clippings***
**Vodka**

Loosely pack the clippings into a large canning jar, and pour in enough vodka to cover them completely. Close the jar tightly and set it in a cool, dark place for 7 to 10 days, shaking it now and then. Strain out the clippings, and pour the liquid into a clean bottle with a tight lid. Dab the chlorophyll on with a cotton ball.

*Don't use clippings from a lawn that's been treated with chemical pesticides.*

## 🍎 LUSCIOUS LIP GLOSS

Here's an easy way to have lip gloss that's your favorite shade *and* your favorite flavor.

**1 tbsp. of petroleum jelly**
**¼ teaspoon of lipstick**
**2–4 drops of flavored extract (e.g., orange, rum, or peppermint)**

Mix all of the ingredients together in a bowl, and scrape the gloss into a small, lidded container. (A clean, empty 35-mm film canister is perfect.)

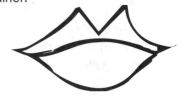

## 🍎 LUXURIOUS BATH OIL

After a long, hard day in the yard (or even a short, easy one), nothing feels better than sinking into a tub full of hot water and this toddy for the body.

**2 cups of milk**
**1 cup of salt**
**1 cup of honey**
**¼ cup of baking soda**
**½ cup of baby oil**

Combine the milk, salt, honey, and baking soda in a large bowl. Fill your bathtub with water, pour in the mixture, and then add the baby oil (and, if you'd like, a few drops of your favorite fragrance).

## MAKE-MINE-MINTY BATH POWDER

If you go for the fresh aroma of mint, here's a bath powder just for you.

**5 tbsp. of talcum powder
1 tbsp. of cornstarch
2 drops of peppermint oil**

Combine all of the ingredients in a bowl, and mix well with a wooden spoon. Pour the mixture into a shaker (like a large salt shaker) or a container with a lid and a big powder puff.

## OATMEAL SCRUB

This bath-time treat cleanses, tones, and softens your skin all over.

**1 cup of dry oatmeal
½ cup of almonds, coarsely ground
1 ripe avocado, peeled and mashed**

Mix the oatmeal and almonds, and put the mixture in a bath mitt or a clean pantyhose foot. Peel the avocado, and mash it in a small bowl. When you're in

the tub or shower, use the filled mitt to scoop up some avocado, and rub it onto your skin. After your bath, rinse, pat dry, and follow with your regular moisturizer.

## OLD-TIME COUGH STOPPER

Got a cough that won't quit? Here's a remedy that works like a charm.

**1 cup of honey
½ cup of olive oil
3–4 tbsp. of lemon juice**

Combine all of the ingredients in a saucepan. Heat for 5 minutes (don't boil), then stir vigorously for 2 minutes. Pour the mixture into a bottle, and take 1 teaspoon every two hours.

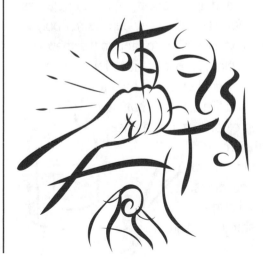

## ▲ OLD-TIME MUSTARD PLASTER

Folks used to treat chest colds, flu, and even pneumonia with this remedy. It still works like a charm—but use it in conjunction with, *not instead of,* your doctor's prescription!

**¼ cup of dry mustard**
**¼ cup of flour**
**3 tbsp. of molasses**
**Thick cream or softened lard**
**Piece of cotton flannel**
**Warm water**

Mix the mustard and flour together, and stir in the molasses. Add enough cream or lard to get an ointment consistency. Dip the cotton flannel in the warm water, wring it out, and lay it on the patient's throat and upper chest, on top of pajamas or a T-shirt, *not against bare skin.* Apply the mixture mixture on top of the the damp cloth, and leave it on for 15 minutes, or until the skin starts to turn red. This stuff is *hot,* so keep close watch and rinse the skin afterwards. If irritation develops, remove the plaster immediately.

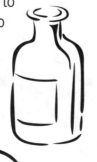

## ▲ OLD-TIME TUMMY TAMER

When nausea strikes, reach for this classic remedy.

**½ cup of fresh-squeezed orange juice**
**2 tbsp. of clear corn syrup**
**Pinch of salt**
**½ cup of water**

Mix all of the ingredients together, and store the potion in a covered jar in the refrigerator. Take 1 tablespoon every half-hour or so until your queasiness has flown the coop.

## ▲ PERFECT PEPPERMINT TOOTHPASTE

This mouth-pleaser will leave your teeth sparklin' clean and make your breath kissin' sweet.

**1 tbsp. of baking soda**
**¼ tsp. of peppermint extract**
**Dash of salt**

Combine the ingredients until you achieve a toothpaste-like consistency. Then brush and enjoy!

## ⚜ PETROLEUM JELLY MUSCLE RELIEVER

Whether your body woes come from long hours on the golf course or a rousing game of Frisbee® with your grandchildren, this simple formula will send your problems packing.

**Warm water**
**Towel**
**1 tbsp. of petroleum jelly**
**6–7 drops of peppermint oil**

Put the towel in warm water to soak. Meanwhile, mix the petroleum jelly and oil in a bowl, and set it in a basin of warm water for about 3 minutes. Wring out the towel, dip it into the oil/jelly mixture, and massage your aching muscles.

## ⚜ REMEDY FOR THE RUNS

Diarrhea is no fun. Fortunately, there's a great-tasting cure.

**1 apple, peeled and cored**
**1 tsp. of lime juice**
**3–4 drops of honey**
**Pinch of cinnamon**

Purée all of the ingredients in a blender, pour the mixture into a bowl, and eat up. Just a few words of caution: Never give this concoction—or anything containing honey—to a baby under 1 year of age. And, if the diarrhea lasts more than a day or two, call your doctor.

## ⚜ SAY "AHHH" MASK

Want a facial that will both soften and invigorate your skin? Just say "Ahhh!" (as in avocado, almonds, and honey).

**2 tbsp. of mashed avocado**
**1 tbsp. of crushed almonds**
**½ tsp. of honey**

Stir all of the ingredients together until the mixture is creamy. Smooth it onto your face with your hands, and leave it for 30 minutes or so. Rinse with warm water and pat dry.

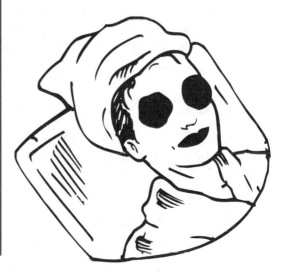

## ⚫ SLEEPY TIME COUGH MEDICINE

When you've got a cough that's keeping you awake at night, reach for this simple sleeping aid.

**1 cup of red wine**
**Lemon**
**Cinnamon**
**Sugar**

Heat the wine (don't let it boil!), and add lemon, cinnamon, and sugar to taste. You'll sleep like a baby!

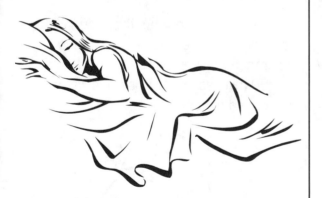

## ⚫ SO-LONG CELLULITE WRAP

Troubled by cellulite? Try this copycat version of the herbal wraps the fancy spas use.

**1 cup of corn oil**
**½ cup of grapefruit juice**
**2 tsp. of dried thyme**

Combine all of the ingredients, and massage the mixture into your thighs, hips, and buttocks. Cover the area with plastic wrap, and hold a heating pad over each body section for 5 minutes.

## ⚫ SORE THROAT GARGLE

When it feels like there's a four-alarm fire raging in your throat, put out the flames with this remedy.

**1 clove of garlic**
**1 tsp. of salt**
**1 tiny pinch of cayenne pepper**
**Water**

Crush the garlic clove and put it into a large glass. Add the salt, pepper, and water, and stir. Then gargle with the solution. Repeat as needed, but if your throat doesn't feel better in a day or so, call your doctor.

## ⚫ SORE THROAT SIPPER

Here's a great-tasting way to ease the pain of a sore throat.

**Juice of 1 lime**
**1 tbsp. of pineapple juice**
**1 tsp. of honey**
**1 glass of water**

Mix the juices and honey in the glass of water, and drink to your health!

## SUPER-SIMPLE BUBBLE BATH

In the mood for a bubble bath? You couldn't find a smoother—or simpler—recipe than this one.

**2 cups of vegetable oil**
**3 tbsp. of mild shampoo**
**¼ tsp. of perfume or scented oil**

Pour all of the ingredients into a blender, blend at high speed, and store in a capped bottle at room temperature. At bath time, pour about ¼ cup of the mixture under running water.

## SUPER-SOOTHING BATH MILK

After a long, hard day, treat yourself to a soak in the tub with this mixture.

**2 cups of powdered milk**
**1 cup of cornstarch**
**2 or 3 drops of your favorite scented oil (optional)**

Mix everything in a blender, and store the mixture in an airtight container at room temperature. At bath time, add ½ cup to a tub of hot water, and enjoy.

## SWEET SALVE

Sugar helps cuts and scrapes heal faster, and lessens the risk of infection by helping to keep the wounds dry. So, the next time you have a minor mishap, slather on some of this healthful salve.

**4 parts sugar**
**1 part Betadine ointment (available in the supermarket's pharmacy or first-aid section)**

First, wash and dry the wound, and make sure it's stopped bleeding (otherwise, the sugar will make it bleed more). Mix the sugar and Betadine together, dab a thick layer onto the cut, and cover it with a bandage. Repeat the procedure three or four times a day in the beginning, decreasing to once a day as healing progresses.

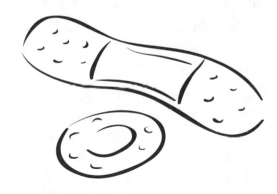

## ☕ TERRIFIC TOOTSIE TREAT

Treat your feet to this terrific tonic.

**1 ripe banana**
**2 tbsp. of honey**
**2 tbsp. of margarine**
**1 tbsp. of lemon juice**

Smash the banana. Then add the rest of the ingredients, and mix until creamy. Massage onto clean, dry feet, paying special attention to any cracked, flaky areas. Pull on a pair of cotton socks, and wear them overnight. (This treatment works for dry hands, too.)

## ☕ THICKENING CONDITIONER

This rich blend will leave your hair looking thicker, shinier, and healthier.

**1 egg yolk**
**½ tsp. of olive oil**
**¾ cup of lukewarm water**

Beat the egg yolk until it's thick and light-colored. Then, as you continue beating, slowly drizzle the oil into the egg. Still beating, slowly add the water. Pour the mixture into a plastic container. After shampooing, massage all of the conditioner into your hair. Leave it on for 3 or 4 minutes, and rinse thoroughly.

## ☕ TOUGH-AS-NAILS TREATMENT

Here's an easy-to-make elixir that will both strengthen and shine your nails.

**2 tsp. of castor oil**
**2 tsp. of salt**
**1 tsp. of wheat germ**

Mix all of the ingredients together, and pour the mixture into a bottle. Shake well before using, and apply it to your nails with a cotton ball.

## ☕ TRIPLE-DUTY FACE CREAM

This triple-treat recipe will remove makeup, and clean and soften your skin.

**½ cup of mayonnaise**
**1 tbsp. of melted butter**
**Juice of 1 lemon or 1 lime**

Mix all of the ingredients together, and store the cream in the refrigerator in a tightly closed glass jar. Use it as you would any facial cleanser, and rinse with cold water.

## ❦ TUTTI-FRUTTI FACIAL

If you like the aroma of a fresh fruit salad, you'll love this softening and invigorating facial.

**6 strawberries**
**½ of an apple**
**½ of a pear**
**1 oz. of orange juice**
**Honey**

Purée the fruits with the orange juice in a blender. Apply a thin layer of honey to your face, then apply the fruit mixture. Leave it on your skin for at least 30 minutes, rinse with warm water, and pat dry.

## ❦ VIOLET CLEANSING MILK

If you like the sweet scent of violets, you'll love this cleanser. It's just the ticket for skin that's dry or sensitive.

**¼ cup of evaporated milk**
**¼ cup of whole milk**
**2 tbsp. of sweet violets, fresh
   or dried**

Put all of the ingredients in the top half of a double boiler, and simmer for about 30 minutes. Don't let the milk boil! Turn off the heat, let the mixture sit for about 2 hours, and strain it into a pretty bottle.

Keep it in the refrigerator. To use the cleanser, pat it onto your face with a cotton ball, massage gently with your fingers, and rinse with cool water.

## ❦ WINE & APPLE MASQUE

Here's a recipe that will slough off dead skin cells, refine your pores, and gradually even out your skin tone.

**2 tbsp. of ground oatmeal***
**2 tsp. of red wine**
**2 tsp. of apple juice**

Mix the oatmeal, wine, and apple juice in small bowl until it forms a spreadable paste (add more liquid if you need to). Smooth the mixture onto your face and neck, and leave it on for 20 to 30 minutes, until dry. Rinse your face with warm water and pat dry.

*Grind the dry oatmeal to a powder in a coffee grinder or blender.*

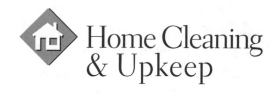

# Home Cleaning & Upkeep

## ◆ ANTI-MOUSE MIX

When mice are driving you crazy, and you don't want to use unpleasant poisons, mix up a batch of this potent alternative.

**1 part flour**
**1 part plaster of Paris**
**Cookie crumbs or powdered chocolate drink mix**

Combine the flour and plaster of Paris, and spoon into shallow containers (jar lids are perfect). Add a pinch or two of cookie crumbs or chocolate drink mix to each lid, and stir it in. Then set out the bait where only mice can get to it (not children or pets), and put a saucer of water nearby.

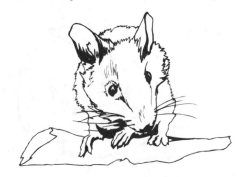

## ◆ BATHROOM MILDEW BANISHER

If cleaning mildew from your tub, glass shower doors, or vinyl curtain liner has become almost a second career, this formula will give you some time off!

**½ cup of rubbing alcohol**
**1 tbsp. of liquid laundry detergent (with enzymes in it)**
**3 cups of water**

Mix all of the ingredients in a hand-held spray bottle, and keep the bottle on the side of the tub. Then make sure that the last person out of the bath or shower each day sprays the solution on all of the wet surfaces. Follow up once a month by wiping down the walls with the same solution, and you should never see mold or mildew again.

## ◆ BRASS AND COPPER POLISH

Here's a recipe that will keep all your brass and copper pieces shipshape enough for an admiral's inspection.

**1 tbsp. of flour**
**1 tbsp. of salt**
**1 tbsp. of white vinegar**

Mix the ingredients to form a thick paste. Apply a generous layer with a damp sponge, gently wiping the metal. Let the polish dry for about an hour, rinse with warm water, and buff with a clean, soft cloth.

## ◆ CHRISTMAS TREE TONIC

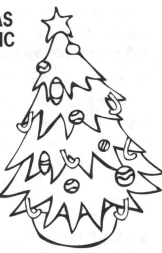

Before you put your Christmas tree on display, give it this pre-treatment to keep it fresh and festive all through the holiday season.

**2 cups of clear corn syrup**
**2 tbsp. of bleach**
**4 multivitamin tablets**
**with iron**
**Very warm water**

Mix the syrup, bleach, and vitamin tablets in a bucket of very warm water. Cut 2 inches off the bottom of the tree's trunk, and stand the tree in the bucket of solution overnight before you put it in its stand. After that, make sure you keep plenty of water in the tree stand at all times.

## ◆ CLOTHESPIN CLEANER

This solution will get dirty, old wooden clothespins as clean as new—and kill any mildew in the process.

**½ cup of bleach**
**1 tbsp. of laundry detergent**
**2 gal. of warm water**

Mix all of the ingredients in a bucket, and soak the clothespins for about 10 minutes. Then pin them on the clothesline to dry in the sun.

## ◆ CRY-NO-MORE MILK CLEANER

Don't cry over spilled milk—or ice cream, either. Instead, clean it off of your upholstery with this fabulous formula.

**Dishwashing liquid**
**2 tbsp. of ammonia**
**Laundry detergent**
**Warm water**

First, scrub the area gently with a mixture of dishwashing liquid and warm water. Follow up with a solution of 2 tablespoons of ammonia in 4 cups of water. Wash the spot again with laundry detergent and water. Finally, saturate a clean cotton cloth with warm water, wring it out, and scrub gently.

## ◆ CUTTING-EDGE CUTTING BOARD CLEANER

Nothing gets a wooden cutting board germ- and odor-free better than this simple formula.

**1 part baking soda**
**1 part salt**
**Water**

Mix the soda and salt with just enough water to make a paste. Scrub this concoction into the board, leave it on for a few hours, and rinse thoroughly.

## ◆ DOWN-HOME DECK CLEANER

Here's the best cleaning formula I've found for wooden decks.

**1 qt. of bleach**
**½ cup of powdered laundry detergent**
**2 gal. of hot water**

Mix all of the ingredients in a bucket. Scrub the deck with a stiff brush (such as a push broom), and then rinse the surface well.

## ◆ DRY CARPET CLEANER

Don't buy dry carpet cleaner—make your own with this simple recipe.

**2 cups of baking soda**
**½ cup of cornstarch**
**1 tbsp. of ground cloves**
**4–5 crumbled bay leaves**

Mix all of the ingredients together, and store the mixture in a shaker jar. (An empty carpet cleaner can is perfect.) To use the mix, dust the carpet thoroughly with the powder, wait at least 1 hour, and then vacuum thoroughly.

## ◆ FABULOUS FURNITURE POLISH

The next time you run out of furniture polish, don't buy more—use this simple, all-natural alternative instead.

**2 tbsp. of lemon juice**
**10 drops of lemon oil**
**4 drops of olive oil**

Mix the juice and the oils in a bowl, dip a soft cotton cloth into the mixture, and apply it gently to your furniture with a circular motion. The potion will nourish the wood and make it smell good, too!

## ◆ GEL AIR FRESHENER

If you like scented air fresheners, you'll love this easy recipe.

**2 cups of distilled water**
**4 cups of unflavored gelatin**
**10–20 drops of fragrance oil**
**Food coloring (optional)**

Heat 1 cup of the water almost to boiling, then add the gelatin and stir until it's dissolved. Remove from the heat and add the remaining cup of water, the fragrance, and the food coloring. Pour the mixture into clean jars, and let them sit at room temperature until they've fully gelled. (They'll set faster in the refrigerator, but be careful—they'll share their scent with your food.)

## ◆ HIGH-POWERED SIDING CLEANER

Get stubborn spots off of vinyl or aluminum siding with this potent formula.

**1 qt. of bleach**
**⅔ cup of TSP***
**⅓ cup of powdered laundry detergent**
**3 qt. of water**

Combine all of the ingredients, and use with a sponge or brush to wash the stains away. Immediately rinse with a garden hose.

*\* Trisodium phosphate, available in hardware stores and many supermarkets.*

## ◆ HOMEMADE DRYER SHEETS

You can make your own dryer sheets and get the same anti-cling power of store-bought kinds, but for a fraction of the cost.

**Liquid fabric softener**
**Water**
**Washcloth**

In a medium-sized mixing bowl, combine 1 part fabric softener and 1 part water. Mix thoroughly. Soak the washcloth in the mix for a minute or two. Wring it out and use it in your dryer to prevent static cling. You can reuse the washcloth several times before laundering it and starting with a new batch of softener.

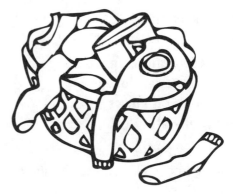

## ◆ HOMEMADE SCOURING POWDER

Here's a simple cleanser that will get grease and grime off of pots and pans, appliances, tile floors, bathroom fixtures, and just about every other surface in— and outside—your house.

**1 cup of baking soda**
**1 cup of borax**
**1 cup of salt**

Combine all of these ingredients, and then store the mixture in a closed container. Use it as you would any powdered cleanser.

## ◆ HOUSE-SALE HELPER

Trying to sell your house? Shortly before potential buyers are due to arrive, put a pot of this elixir on the stove. Real estate surveys show that its spicy-sweet aroma is one of the two most likely to make house-hunters think, "This is the place!" (The other is fresh-baked bread.)

**Rind of 1 orange, shaved**
**¼ cup of whole cloves**
**4–5 cinnamon sticks**
**3–4 qt. of water**

Bring a pot of water to boiling, and add the orange peel, cloves, and cinnamon sticks. Let the brew simmer until the scent has wafted through the house (or at least the kitchen), then turn off the heat.

## ◆ NO-RINSE, ALL-PURPOSE CLEANER

Who needs expensive, "miracle" spray cleaners? This old-time recipe cleans floors, woodwork, greasy countertops, and appliances, and even kills mildew. What's more, you don't even need to rinse!

**1 cup of clear ammonia**
**½ cup of white vinegar**
**¼ cup of baking soda**
**1 gal. of hot water**

Mix all of the ingredients in a bucket. Then pour the solution into a hand-held spray bottle, or sponge it on straight from the pail.

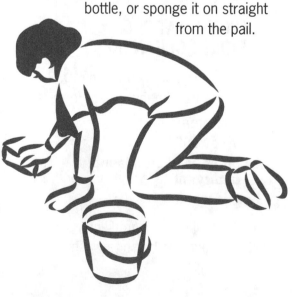

## ◆ NO-STICK, NO-STAIN FORMULA

Get stains off of non-stick pans with this mix.

**3 tbsp. of oxygen bleach made**
**    for delicate fabrics**
**1 tsp. of dishwashing liquid**
**1 cup of water**
**Vegetable oil**

Combine the bleach, dishwashing liquid, and water. Pour the mixture into the stained pan, and simmer until the stains vanish. Then wash the pan, dry it thoroughly, and coat it lightly with the vegetable oil.

## ◆ ONE-SHOT CLEANER

Here's a great recipe for a multipurpose cleaner that works like magic!

**2 cups of rubbing alcohol**
**1 tbsp. of ammonia**
**1 tbsp. of dishwashing liquid**
**2 qt. of water**

Mix the ingredients, pour the solution into a hand-held spray bottle, and go to town. (Incidentally, this super-duper concoction will beat commercial, streakless glass-cleaning products hands down!)

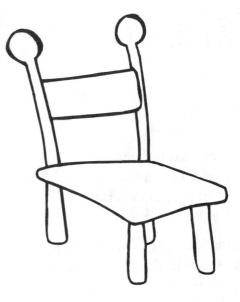

## ◆ PERFECT POLISH FOR WOOD

Here's a great furniture polish for any kind of wood furniture.

**½ cup of linseed oil**
**¼ cup of malt vinegar**
**1 tsp. of lemon or lavender oil**

Put the linseed oil and vinegar in a clean jar with a tight lid, and shake it vigorously. Stir in the lemon or lavender oil. Apply it to your furniture with a clean, soft cotton cloth, and buff with a second, clean cloth. (In hot, humid weather, reverse the proportions, so that you're combining ¼ cup of linseed oil and ½ cup of vinegar, because damp heat tends to make oil, well, oilier.)

## ◆ SAFE & SOUND DRAIN CLEANER

Use this unclogger once a month to keep your drains open and clean-smelling—without corroding your plumbing or burning your skin.

**⅓ cup of baking soda**
**⅓ cup of table salt**
**1 tbsp. of cream of tartar**
**1 cup of boiling water**

Combine the soda, salt, and cream of tartar, and pour the mixture into the drain. Immediately add 1 cup of boiling water. Wait 10 seconds, then flush with cold water for at least 20 seconds.

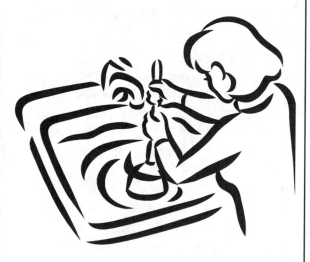

## ◆ STICK 'EM TO IT FLYPAPER

When fly season rolls around, don't reach for a spray gun. Make up a batch of good old-fashioned flypaper instead.

**1 cup of corn syrup**
**1 tbsp. of brown sugar**
**1 tbsp. of white sugar**
**1 brown paper bag**

Cut the bag into strips about 1 inch wide. Poke a hole in the top of each one, and put a string through it. Then mix the syrup and the sugar together, brush the gooey stuff onto the strips, and hang them wherever flies are bugging you.

## ◆ SUPER SILVER CLEANING FORMULA

Here's the easiest recipe I know of for getting tarnished silver bright, shiny, and new-looking again.

**Aluminum foil**
**2 pans that can hold enough water to cover your silver piece**
**1 cup of baking soda per gal. of water**
**Water**

Line the bottom of one pan with foil, and set your tarnished treasure in it. Make sure the silver touches the aluminum (I say this in case there's a non-silver part

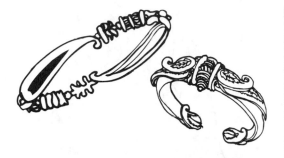

to the object). Then fill the second pan with water and heat it to boiling. Remove the pan from the heat, set it in the sink, and add the baking soda. Be careful—the solution will foam up and may spill over. Pour the soda solution into the first pan, completely covering the silver. Within seconds, you'll see the tarnish start to disappear. A lightly tarnished piece should be clean-as-a-whistle in 4 or 5 minutes; one with a heavy coat of tarnish may need a few more treatments.

## ◆ TIME-FOR-TEA CLEANSER

Don't throw away your leftover tea leaves. Instead, save them to make this homemade cleanser.

**1 cup of black tea leaves**
**1 tsp. of baking soda**
**3–4 drops of dishwashing liquid**

Combine all of the ingredients, and use the stuff for general cleaning as you would any scouring powder. To clean your oven, heat the mixture, and wipe it all over your oven. Let it sit for a few minutes, scrub with a brush or sponge, and rinse with warm water. For pans that are caked with burned-on food, put the mixture inside, and heat it. Remove the pan from the heat, wipe the mixture over the surface, and let it sit for a few minutes. Scrub with a scouring sponge, pour the cleanser out, and wash the pan in warm, soapy water.

## ◆ ULTIMATE RANGE CLEANER

When your stove top is covered in spaghetti sauce splatters and who-knows-what-else, reach for this remedy.

**3 tbsp. of salt**
**3 tbsp. of baking soda**
**Pinch of cream of tartar**
**Hydrogen peroxide**

Combine the baking soda, salt, and cream of tartar in a bowl. Add enough hydrogen peroxide to make a paste. Spread this concoction on the stains and let it sit for a half-hour or so, then scrub with a sponge dipped in warm water.

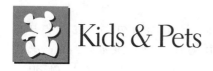

# Kids & Pets

## ■ BATHTUB COOKIES

These bath-time "cookies" are the perfect bribe for reluctant young bathers. They also make great gifts.

**2 cups of fine-grain sea salt\***
**½ cup of cornstarch**
**½ cup of baking soda**
**2 tbsp. of light vegetable oil**
**1 tsp. of vitamin E oil**
**6 drops of your favorite scented oil**
**6 drops of food coloring (optional)**

Mix all of the ingredients together, roll out the dough, and cut out shapes with cookie cutters. Bake at 350°F for 10 to 12 minutes. (Don't overbake!) Let the cookies cool completely, and put them in a big glass jar or other decorative container. To use, just add one or two cookies to the bathwater, and enjoy!

*\* If your supermarket doesn't have fine-grain sea salt, use kosher salt instead, and run it through your blender or coffee grinder.*

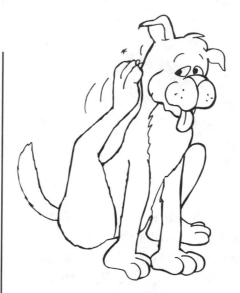

## ■ FLEE, FLEAS LEMON RINSE

Here's a pet-pleasing rinse that will help keep felines and canines flea-free all summer long.

**1 lemon, thinly sliced**
**1 qt. of hot water**

Put the lemon slices in the water, and let the brew steep overnight. Once a day during flea season, groom your pet with a flea comb, then sponge on the lemon rinse. Note: Test it on a small patch of your pet's skin first—some cats and dogs are allergic to the oils in citrus fruits.

## ■ FROZEN BIRD TREATS

Want to give your pet bird a cool and healthy treat? Whip up a batch of these goodies.

1 qt. (32 oz.) of vanilla yogurt
1 cup of mashed fruit*
2 tbsp. of peanut butter
2 tbsp. of honey

Mix all of the ingredients in a blender, and freeze the mixture in ice cube trays or, for larger birds, 3-ounce paper cups. Then, when Polly wants a snack, pop one into the microwave, nuke it for a few seconds, and serve it up.

* Or substitute 1 large jar of baby fruit.

## ■ FUN & FANCY SOAP

Kids and grownups alike will love this colorful, easy-to-make soap.

1 bar of floating bath soap (such as Ivory®), grated
4–6 drops of food coloring
2–3 drops of flavored extract
¼ cup of warm water

Mix all of the ingredients in a bowl until stiff. Remove from the bowl, and knead to the consistency of very thick dough. Spoon into plastic molds or cookie cutters and set in the freezer for 10 minutes. Pop the soaps out of the molds, and let dry until hard.

## ■ HOMEMADE BABY WIPES

Why buy expensive baby wipes when you've probably got everything you need to make your own? Here's how it's done.

1 roll of soft, absorbent paper towels (premium brands work best)
1 plastic container with tight-fitting lid to hold the paper towels
2 tbsp. of baby oil
2 tbsp. of liquid baby bath soap
2 cups of water

Cut the roll of paper towels in half with a serrated knife, and remove the cardboard tube. Place half the roll, on end, in the plastic container. Mix the liquid ingredients, pour the solution into the container, and close the lid. The towels will absorb the liquid. As you need them, pull the wipes up from the center of the roll.

## ■ HOMEMADE FINGER PAINTS

Treat your budding artist to these custom-made paints.

**¼ cup of cornstarch**
**2 cups of cold water**
**Food coloring**

Combine the cornstarch and water in a pan, and boil, stirring constantly, until the mixture thickens. Pour it into small containers, and add the food coloring of your choice to each one. (The more you add, of course, the darker the paint will be.)

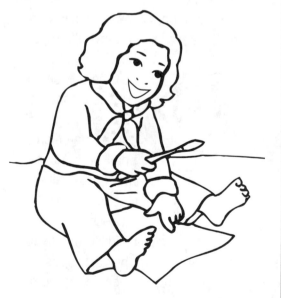

## ■ LET'S-GIVE-A-SHOW MAKEUP

When Halloween rolls around, or it's time for a pint-sized dramatic production, make up some makeup for your young superstars.

**2 tbsp. of cornstarch**
**1 tbsp. of solid shortening**
**Food coloring (optional)**

Mix the cornstarch and shortening together, and stir in whatever food coloring the role calls for. (Omit the food coloring for plain white clowns and scary ghosts!)

## ■ NO-FLAME FORMULA

Fire departments recommend this recipe for making children's clothes (or any other fabric) flame-retardant.

**9 oz. of borax**
**4 oz. of boric acid**
**1 gal. of water**

Mix all of the ingredients together. Spray the solution onto non-washable fabrics. To treat washable items, launder as usual, soak them in the solution after the final rinse, then dry. To be on the safe side, repeat the treatment after each washing or dry cleaning.

# ■ PLAYFUL DOUGH

The young sculptors in your life will have a ball with this homemade playdough.

**2 cups of flour**
**4 tbsp. of cream of tartar**
**2 tbsp. of vegetable oil**
**1 cup of table salt**
**3–4 drops of food coloring**
**2 cups of water**

Combine all of the ingredients in a saucepan, and stir over medium heat for 3 to 5 minutes, until the mixture forms a ball. When it cools, mix it with your hands, and let the fun begin! Store in an airtight container.

# ■ PUP-SICLES

For hot-weather treats—or to distract a teething puppy from your favorite sneakers—gather some ice cube trays, and make batches of these goodies.

**½ cup of finely chopped**
**    vegetables**
**½ cup of plain yogurt**
**1 qt. of beef or chicken bouillon**

Mix all of the ingredients together, and pour the mixture into ice cube trays. Then tuck them into the freezer until treat time rolls around.

# ■ SOOTHING SUNBURN BATH

Kids love this foaming bath, even when they don't have sunburned skin. (Grownups go for it, too.)

**1 cup of vegetable oil**
**½ cup of honey**
**½ cup of liquid hand soap**
**1 tbsp. of pure vanilla extract**
**    (not artificial)**

Mix all of the ingredients together, and pour the mixture into a bottle with a tight stopper. At bath time, shake the bottle, then pour ¼ cup under running water.

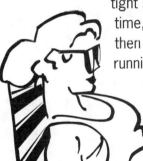

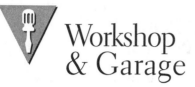

## Workshop & Garage

## ▼ ALL-PURPOSE CLEANUP MIX

Here's a handy recipe that you can use on stucco, concrete, or any other outdoor surface.

⅓ **cup of powdered laundry detergent**
⅔ **cup of powdered household detergent, like Spic and Span®**
1 **gal. of water**

Mix all of the ingredients together, put on a pair of rubber gloves, grab a sponge, and you're ready to go. Use a stiff-bristle brush to scrub stubborn stains. If you're

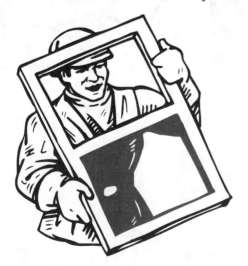

cleaning something that's mildewed, use less water and add about a pint of bleach to the mix.

## ▼ LIME-BE-GONE SOLUTION

This simple recipe will get rid of lime and hard-water deposits on flowerpots, water spigots, or anything else, indoors or out.

½ **cup of borax**
1 **cup of warm water**
½ **cup of white vinegar**

Dissolve the borax in the water, and stir in the vinegar. Sponge the solution onto the lime deposits, let it sit for 10 minutes or so (longer for really stubborn spots), and wipe clean.

## ▼ SEE-THE-LIGHT SOLUTION

When your car's headlights—or taillights—get so grimy you can hardly see their beams, reach for this recipe.

2 **tbsp. of ammonia**
1 **tbsp. of cornstarch**
1 **qt. of water**

Mix all of the ingredients together in a bucket, dip a sponge into the liquid, and wash the grease and grime away. Rinse with clear water.

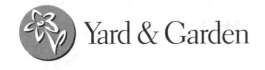 Yard & Garden

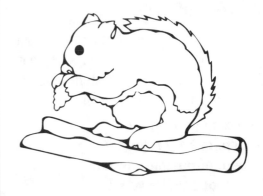

## ● ALL-AROUND DISEASE DEFENDER

When cool, damp weather strikes, protect your plants from fungal diseases with this classic defense mix.

**1 cup of chamomile tea**
**1 tsp. of dishwashing liquid**
**½ tsp. of vegetable oil**
**½ tsp. of peppermint oil**
**1 gal. of warm water**

Mix all of the ingredients in a bucket. Mist-spray your plants every week or so when temperatures are below 75°F.

## ● ALL-PURPOSE VARMINT REPELLENT

No matter what kind of four-legged felons are invading your garden, this classic tonic will send them packing.

**2 eggs**
**2 cloves of garlic**
**2 tbsp. of hot chile pepper**
**2 tbsp. of ammonia**
**2 cups of water**

Combine all of the ingredients, and let the mixture sit for 3 or 4 days. Then paint it on fences, trellises, and wherever else unwelcome critters are venturing.

## ● ANNUAL PICK-ME-UP TONIC

In late summer, when your annuals seem on the brink of exhaustion, give them a dose of this energizer.

**¼ cup of beer**
**1 tbsp. of corn syrup**
**1 tbsp. of baby shampoo**
**1 tbsp. of 15-30-15 fertilizer**
**1 gal. of water**

Mix all of these ingredients in a watering can, and slowly dribble the solution onto the root zones of your plants.

## ● ANT AMBROSIA

Here's a formula that's lethal to ants, but won't harm kids or pets. (Fido will love it, though, so if you want the stuff to do its duty, keep it out of his reach!)

**4–5 tbsp. of cornmeal**
**3 tbsp. of bacon grease**
**3 tbsp. of baking powder**
**3 pkg. of baker's yeast**

Mix the cornmeal and bacon grease into a paste, then add the baking powder and yeast. Dab the gooey mix on the sides of jar lids, and set them out in your invaded territory. Ants will love it to death!

## ● ANT ANNIHILATOR

When ants are driving you nuts, use this ultimate weapon.

**1 part flour**
**1 part sugar**
**1 part borax**
**1 part alum**
**Water**

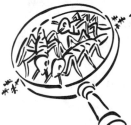

Mix the dry ingredients with just enough water to make a batter. Pour into shallow pans, and set them out where the ants congregate. Just make sure that children, pets, and other non-ants can't get at it!

## ● ANT-ICIDE

If ants are on the brink of taking over your kitchen, this'll stop 'em dead in their tracks.

**2 parts molasses**
**1 part sugar**
**1 part dry yeast powder**

Mix all of the ingredients together, spoon a little of the goo onto pieces of paper, and then set them all around in the problem areas.

## ● BASIC OIL MIXTURE

Scale insects and a whole lot of other pests go belly-up when they strike oil—or rather, when oil strikes *them!*

**1 cup of vegetable oil**
**1 tbsp. of Murphy's Oil Soap®**

Pour the oil and the oil soap into a plastic squeeze bottle, and store at room temperature. To use, put 1 tablespoon of the mixture in 2 cups of water in a hand-held spray bottle, and spray your pest-ridden plants from top to bottom. (Shake the bottle now and then to make sure the oil and water stay mixed.)

## ● BRUSSELS SPROUTS ELIXIR

If you're looking for a nontoxic herbicide for annual weeds, this recipe's for you. Use in early spring, before the seeds germinate.

(The secret ingredient, in the Brussels sprouts, is thiocyanate, a chemical that's toxic to newly germinated seeds.)

**2 cups of Brussels sprouts**
**Water**
**½ tsp. of dishwashing liquid**

In a blender, mix the Brussels sprouts with enough water to make a thick mush. Add ½ teaspoon of dishwashing liquid, and pour the mix into cracks in your sidewalk or driveway, or anyplace you want to stop weeds before they germinate. (Be careful where you use this: Thiocyanate won't hurt established plants, but it can't tell the difference between seeds you've sown, or volunteers you're hoping for, and weeds you want to get rid of!)

## ● BULB BATH

To keep your bulbs healthy and bug-free, treat them to this nice, warm bath before tucking them into their planting bed.

**2 tsp. of baby shampoo**
**1 tsp. of antiseptic mouthwash**
**¼ tsp. of instant tea granules**
**2 gal. of warm water**

Mix all of the ingredients in a bucket, and carefully set your bulbs into the solution. Stir gently, then remove the bulbs one at a time and plant them. When you're through,

serve the nutritious bathwater to a thirsty tree or shrub.

## ● BULB-CLEANING TONIC

In the fall, when you dig up your tender bulbs, wash them in this tonic.

**2 tbsp. of baby shampoo**
**1 tsp. of hydrogen peroxide**
**1 qt. of warm water**

Mix all of these ingredients together, and give your bulbs a warm bath. Make sure you dry the bulbs thoroughly before you store them for winter, or else they'll rot.

## ● BYE BYE BLACK SPOT SPRAY

This simple formula works like a charm to head off black spot on roses.

**1 tbsp. of baking soda**
**1 tsp. of dishwashing liquid**
**1 gal. of water**

Mix these ingredients together, pour the solution into a hand-held spray bottle, and spray your roses every three days during the growing season. There'll be no more singin' the black spot blues!

## ● COMPOST BOOSTER TONIC

Keep your compost pile cooking up a storm with this tonic.

**1 can of regular cola (not diet)**
**1 can of beer**
**1 cup of dishwashing liquid**

Combine all of the ingredients in your 20 gallon hose-end sprayer, and spray your compost pile once a month.

## ● CONTAINER PLANT STARTER

Get your outdoor container plants off to a great start with this healthful soil booster.

**2 cups dry oatmeal**
**2 cups dry dog food, crushed**
**Pinch of human hair\***
**1½ tsp. of sugar**

Combine all of these ingredients, and add 2 tablespoons of the mixture to moistened, professional potting soil for each container.

*\* Ask your hair stylist or barber for discarded hair cuttings.*

## ● CONTAINER PLANT TONIC

To water your outdoor container plants, make this marvelous master mix of fortified feed.

**1 tbsp. of 15-30-15 fertilizer**
**½ tsp. of gelatin powder**
**½ tsp. of dishwashing liquid**
**½ tsp. of corn syrup**
**½ tsp. of whiskey**
**¼ tsp. of instant tea granules**
**Water**

Mix the first six ingredients in a 1-gallon milk jug, and fill the balance of the jug with water. Stir, and add ½ cup of the mixture to every gallon of water you use to water your container plants.

## ● DAYLILY TRANSPLANT TONIC

When you divide daylilies or other perennial favorites, get the transplanted divisions off to a good start with this elixir.

**½ can of beer**
**2 tbsp. of dishwashing liquid**
**2 tbsp. of ammonia**
**2 tbsp. of Fish Emulsion (a fertilizer available at garden centers)**
**1 tbsp. of hydrogen peroxide**
**¼ tsp. of instant tea granules**
**2 gal. of water**

Mix all of these ingredients in a large bucket. Just before setting the plants into their new homes, pour 2 cups of the mixture into each hole.

## ● DOG-BE-GONE TONIC

Keep roaming dogs out of your yard with this spicy potion.

**2 cloves of garlic**
**2 small onions**
**1 jalapeño pepper**
**1 tbsp. of cayenne pepper**
**1 tbsp. of Tabasco® sauce**
**1 tbsp. of chili powder**
**1 tbsp. of dishwashing liquid**
**1 qt. of warm water**

Chop the garlic, onions, and pepper, and combine them with the rest of the ingredients. Let the mixture sit for 24 hours, then strain out the solids and sprinkle the solution on any areas where dogs are a problem.

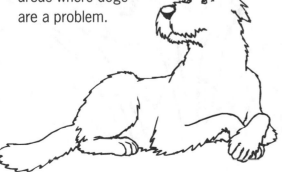

## ● FAIRY RING FIGHTER TONIC

Fairy ring (rings of mushrooms) will vanish from your lawn if you follow this simple recipe.

**2 cups of dry laundry soap (not detergent)**
**1 cup of baby shampoo**
**1 cup of antiseptic mouthwash**
**1 cup of ammonia**

Sprinkle the laundry detergent on the troubled area, and water it in well. Then mix the other ingredients in your 20 gallon hose-end sprayer, and apply it to the point of run-off.

## ● FLOURISHING FERN TONIC

When your ferns are ailing, give 'em what your grandma gave you: a dose of castor oil. Here's the recipe.

**1 tbsp. of castor oil**
**1 tbsp. of baby shampoo**
**1 qt. of warm water**

Combine all of the ingredients in a pail or watering can, and give each plant ¼ cup of the solution. They'll turn green and fresh almost overnight.

## ● FLOWER FEEDER TONIC

This healthy mix of supermarket products includes potent doses of all of the "Big Three" plant nutrients (nitrogen, phosphorus, and potassium) plus essential trace minerals—in other words, everything your perennials need to churn out beautiful blossoms, year after year.

**1 can of beer**
**2 tbsp. of Fish Emulsion (a fertilizer available at garden centers)**
**2 tbsp. of dishwashing liquid**
**2 tbsp. of ammonia**
**2 tbsp. of hydrogen peroxide**
**2 tbsp. of whiskey**
**1 tbsp. of clear corn syrup**
**1 tbsp. of unflavored gelatin powder**
**4 tsp. of instant tea granules**
**2 gal. of warm water**

Mix all of the ingredients together in a large bucket, and feed all of your perennials with the solution every two weeks during the growing season.

## ● FLOWER GARDEN NIGHTCAP

When it's time to close up your flower beds for the season, cover them with finely mowed grass clippings, and overspray with this elixir.

**1 can of regular cola**
**1 cup of baby shampoo**
**½ cup of ammonia**
**2 tbsp. of instant tea granules**

Mix all of these ingredients in your 20 gallon hose-end sprayer, and saturate the grass-clipping blanket.

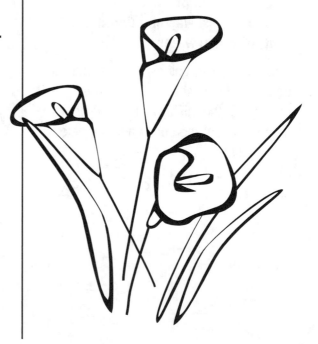

# ● FLOWERING HOUSEPLANT TONIC

Your flowering houseplants will bloom to beat the band if you give them a dose of this elixir every two weeks or so.

½ tbsp. of vodka
½ tbsp. of ammonia
½ tbsp. of hydrogen peroxide
¼ tsp. of instant tea granules
1 multivitamin tablet with iron
1 gal. of warm water

Mix all of the ingredients together in a jug. Add 1 cup of the solution per gallon of water at plant-feeding time. (For non-flowering plants, replace the vodka with ½ tablespoon of bourbon.)

# ● FLOWERING PLANT FOOD

This nutritious mix makes a great meal for any flowering plant.

2 cups dry oatmeal
2 cups dry dog food, crushed
1 part human hair*

Combine all of these ingredients in a bucket, and work the mixture into the soil every two to three weeks during the growing season.

* You can ask your hair stylist or barber for discarded hair cuttings.

# ● FLOWER-SAVER SOLUTION

Make your cut flowers last longer by filling your vases with this libation. This recipe makes 1 quart of solution.

1 cup of lemon-lime soda (not diet)
¼ tsp. of bleach
3 cups of warm water (110°F)

Mix all of these ingredients together, and pour the solution into a clean vase. It'll keep those posies perky and bright.

# ● FUNGUS-FIGHTER SOIL DRENCH

This strong stuff is just the ticket for fighting soil-borne fungi in your garden.

4 garlic bulbs, crushed
½ cup of baking soda
1 gal. of water

Combine all of the ingredients in a pan. Bring the water to a boil. Turn off the heat, and let it cool to room temperature. Strain the liquid into a watering can, and soak the ground around fungus-prone plants. Go *very* slowly, so the liquid goes deep down into the soil. Then gently work the strained-out garlic into the soil.

## ● FUNGUS-FIGHTER TONIC

This terrific tonic works like magic to fend off fungi on ornamental and edible plants.

**½ cup of molasses**
**½ cup of powdered milk**
**1 tsp. of baking soda**
**1 gal. of warm water**

Mix the molasses, powdered milk, and baking soda into a paste. Place the mixture into an old pantyhose leg, and let it steep in the warm water for several hours. Strain, pour the remaining liquid into a hand-held spray bottle, and spritz your fungus-prone plants every week or so during the growing season.

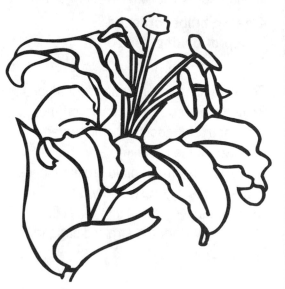

## ● GARLIC AND ONION JUICE

This aromatic elixir controls pests on fruit, flower, or vegetable plants.

**2 cloves of garlic**
**2 medium onions**
**3 cups of water**

Put all of the ingredients in a blender, and whirl them up. Strain out the solids, pour the remaining liquid into a hand-held spray bottle, and use it whenever you need potent relief from soft-bodied insects. Bury the leftover solids in your garden to repel aphids and any other pesky pests.

## ● GARLIC OIL

Mix up this concentrate, and reach for it when you need to solve big-time bug problems.

**1 whole bulb of garlic, minced**
**1 cup of vegetable oil**

Mix the garlic and oil together in a glass jar with a tight lid. Put the mixture in the refrigerator to steep for a day or two, then test it for "doneness." If your eyes don't water when you open the lid, add another half-bulb of minced garlic, and wait another day. Strain out the solids, and pour the oil into a fresh jar. Keep it in the fridge until you're ready to use it. Dilute it as indicated in any recipe that calls for garlic oil.

## ● GO, GERANIUMS! TONIC

Get your geraniums off to a rip-roaring start with this terrific tonic.

**Epsom salts**
**1 cup of beer**
**¼ cup of instant tea granules**
**2 tsp. of baby shampoo**
**1 gal. of water**

Sprinkle the soil with 1 tablespoon of Epsom salts for each 4 inches of pot size. Then mix the remaining ingredients together, and use the mix to water the salts into the soil around your plants.

## ● GO HOME, PETS! TONIC

Keep neighborhood dogs and cats off of your lawn with this simple solution.

**2–3 garlic cloves**
**3–4 hot peppers**
**2–3 drops of dishwashing liquid**
**2 gal. of water**

Purée the garlic and peppers in a blender, then mix them with the dishwashing liquid and water. Dribble the

elixir around the edges of your lawn and sidewalk. Repeat frequently, especially after each rain.

## ● GOPHER-GO TONIC

Got gophers that won't give up? So did I—until I came up with this absolutely amazing recipe.

**4 tbsp. of castor oil**
**4 tbsp. of dishwashing liquid**
**4 tbsp. of urine**
**½ cup of warm water**
**2 gal. of warm water**

Combine the oil, dishwashing liquid, and urine in ½ cup of warm water, then stir the solution into 2 gallons of warm water. Pour the mixture over problem areas, and the gophers will go—fast!

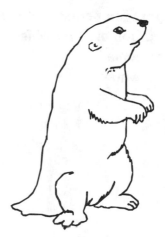

## GRASS SEED STARTER TONIC

This nifty little tonic will guarantee almost 100% germination every time!

**¼ cup of baby shampoo**
**1 tbsp. of Epsom salts**
**1 gal. of weak tea**

Mix all of these ingredients together. Drop in your grass seed, and put the container in the refrigerator for at least 24 hours. Spread the seeds out on your driveway to dry, and sow them in the usual way.

## HAPPY HERB TONIC

Keep your herb garden healthy and productive with this elixir.

**1 cup of tea**
**½ tbsp. of hydrogen peroxide**
**½ tbsp. of bourbon or other whiskey**
**½ tbsp. of ammonia**
**1 gal. of warm water**

Mix all of the ingredients together in a bucket, and feed your herb plants with the solution every six weeks throughout the growing season.

## HEALTHY HOUSEPLANT TONIC

To keep your houseplants in the pink of health, feed them with this elixir.

**1 can of apple juice**
**1 can of beer**
**1 can of regular cola (not diet)**
**1 cup of lemon-scented dishwashing liquid**
**1 cup of lemon-scented ammonia**
**½ cup of Fish Emulsion (a fertilizer available at garden centers)**

Mix all of these ingredients in a big old pot. Store the solution in a covered container, and use 3 ounces per gallon of water every other time you water your houseplants.

## ● HERB BOOSTER TONIC

When the weather turns steamy, even herbs enjoy a cool drink. Quench their thirst with this summertime pick-me-up.

**1 can of beer**
**1 cup of ammonia**
**½ cup of corn syrup**
**½ cup of Murphy's Oil Soap®**

Mix all of these ingredients in your 20 gallon hose-end sprayer, and spray your herbs every six weeks during the growing season.

## ● HOLIDAY HOUSEPLANT TONIC

Your holiday houseplants will stay chipper all season long if you feed them with this solution.

**¼ cup of beer**
**½ tbsp. of unflavored gelatin powder**
**½ tbsp. of Fish Emulsion (a fertilizer available at garden centers)**
**½ tbsp. of Vitamin B$_1$ Plant Starter**
**½ tbsp. of ammonia**
**½ tbsp. of instant tea granules**
**1 gal. of water**

Mix all of these ingredients together, and use the solution every time you water your holiday plants.

## ● HOMEMADE BIRD TREATS

Your fine feathered friends will flock to your feeder when you serve up this gourmet chow.

**1 part cornmeal**
**1 part wild-bird seed**
**Bacon grease (room-temperature)**
**2 pinches of sand or crushed eggshells**

Mix the cornmeal and bird seed with enough bacon grease to get a bread-dough consistency. Add the sand or eggshells. Shape the dough into a ball, put it in a mesh onion bag, and hang it from a sturdy tree branch or bird-feeder post.

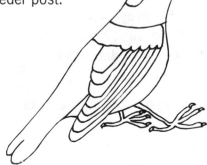

## ● HOUSEPLANT COLORIZER

Here's a simple formula that will keep your houseplants at their peak of color.

**1 twice-used tea bag**
**3 drops of antiseptic mouthwash**
**3 drops of mild shampoo**
**3 drops of ammonia**
**1 quart of water**

Combine all of these ingredients, and let the mixture steep for about 10 minutes. Fish out the tea bag, pour the liquid into a hand-held sprayer, and mist your plants' foliage every week or so.

## ● HOUSEPLANT FOLIAGE TONIC

Your houseplants will have the healthiest, lushest foliage in town if you feed them with this elixir.

**½ tbsp. of bourbon or other whiskey**
**½ tbsp. of ammonia**
**½ tbsp. of hydrogen peroxide**
**¼ tsp. of instant tea granules**
**1 multivitamin tablet with iron**
**1 gal. of warm water**

Mix all of these ingredients together, and water your plants with the solution every week or so.

## ● HURRY-UP-THE-HARVEST TONIC

When Old Man Winter is coming in fast, and your garden is still full of unripe veggies, give your plants a drink of this pungent elixir.

**1 cup of apple juice**
**½ cup of ammonia**
**½ cup of baby shampoo**
**Warm water**

Mix all of the ingredients in your 20 gallon hose-end sprayer jar. Fill the balance of the jar with warm water, and spray your plants to the point of run-off.

## ● INSTANT ANTIQUE TONIC

Want to give your flowerpots an antique look? You can—here's the easy recipe.

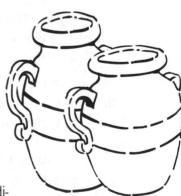

**½ can of beer**
**1 cup of moss**
**½ tsp. of sugar**

Mix all of the ingredients on low speed in a blender. Then paint the mixture on the outside of your containers. In a week or so, moss and lichen will start to form.

## ● INSTANT INSECTICIDE

When there's no time to fumble with fancy formulas, mix up this potent pest killer. It's instant death to almost any bad bug in the book.

**1 cup of rubbing alcohol**
**1 tsp. of vegetable oil**
**1 qt. of water**

Mix all of the ingredients in a hand-held spray bottle, take aim, and give each pest a direct hit.

## ● LAWN FOOD MIX

Whenever you feed your lawn, use this surefire formula.

**3 lb. of Epsom salts**
**1 cup of dry laundry detergent**
**1 bag of dry lawn food (enough to cover 2,500 square feet)**

Mix all of these ingredients together, and apply at half the recommended rate with your hand-held broadcast spreader.

## ● LAWN FRESH-UP TONIC

How do you know when to water your grass? Simple: Walk on it. If it doesn't spring right back up, it's thirsty. To help the water go straight to the roots, put on your golf shoes or a pair of aerating lawn sandals, and take a stroll around your yard. Then follow up with this tonic.

**1 can of beer**
**1 cup of baby shampoo**
**½ cup of ammonia**
**½ cup of weak tea**

Mix all of these ingredients in your 20 gallon hose-end sprayer, and apply until the point of run-off.

## ● LAWN STARTER TONIC

Putting in a new lawn? Get it off to a trouble-free start with this recipe.

**1 cup of Fish Emulsion (a fertilizer available at garden centers)**
**½ cup of ammonia**
**¼ cup of baby shampoo**
**¼ cup of clear corn syrup**

Mix all of these ingredients in your 20 gallon hose-end sprayer, and saturate the soil. Wait several days before you sow the seed.

## ● LETHAL LEAF-EATER SPRAY

This potent potion will bid *adieu* to all kinds of leaf-eating bugs.

**4–6 garlic cloves**
**2 hot peppers***
**1 small onion**
**1 qt. of water**
**3 drops of baby shampoo**

Put the garlic, peppers, and onion in a blender with the water, and liquefy. Let it sit overnight, strain out the solids, and add the baby shampoo. Pour the solution into a hand-held spray bottle, and when the enemy comes into view, let 'em have it!

* *Or 1 teaspoon of ground cayenne.*

## ● LIME-BE-GONE SOLUTION

This simple recipe will get rid of lime and hard-water deposits on flowerpots, water spigots, or anything else, indoors or out.

**½ cup of borax**
**1 cup of warm water**
**½ cup of white vinegar**

Dissolve the borax in the water, and stir in the vinegar. Sponge the mix onto the lime deposits, let it sit for 10 minutes or

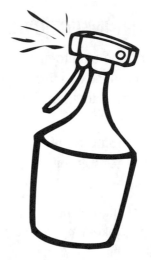

so (longer for really stubborn spots), and wipe clean.

## ● MILDEW RELIEF TONIC

Protect your roses and other mildew-prone plants by spraying them every week in the spring with this fabulous formula.

**1 tbsp. of hydrogen peroxide**
**1 tbsp. of baby shampoo**
**1 tsp. of instant tea granules**
**2 cups of water**

Mix all of these ingredients in a hand-held sprayer, and mist your plants' leaves thoroughly. Mid-afternoon on a cloudy day is the best time to do the job.

## ● MITE-FREE FRUIT TREE FORMULA

Mites might be teeny, but they can do BIG damage to fruit trees. When the pests attack, protect your crop with this easy recipe.

**5 lb. of white flour**
**1 pt. of buttermilk**
**25 gal. of water**

Mix all of the ingredients together, and keep the potion in a tightly closed garbage can. Stir before use, and spray weekly until the mites are history.

## ● MOSS-GROW TONIC

Here's an easy recipe for making moss grow between stepping stones in a path, or on the sides of a planter.

**½ qt. of buttermilk**
**1 cup of moss**
**1 tsp. of corn syrup**

Mix all of the ingredients in a blender, then dab the mixture onto the ground or the sides of the planter. Once the moss is growing, keep it in good health by "watering" it with plain buttermilk every few weeks.

## ● NO-MORE-FLIES FORMULA

Fly troubles will be a thing of the past when you serve up this concoction.

**1 egg yolk**
**1 tbsp. of molasses**
**Pinch of black pepper**

Beat the egg yolk with the molasses and pepper, and pour the mixture into jar lids or shallow cans. The flies will fly in for a three-point landing, but they won't be able to take off again.

## ● PEPPERMINT SOAP SPRAY

When you need to go after hard-bodied bugs like beetles and weevils, you can't find a better weapon than this.

**2 tbsp. of dishwashing liquid**
**2 tsp. of peppermint oil**
**1 gal. of warm water**

Mix all of these ingredients together. Then pour the solution into a hand-held spray bottle, take aim, and fire.

## ● POLLUTION SOLUTION TONIC

Dust, dirt, and pollution accumulate on your lawn over the winter, causing it to look like a heck of a wreck in spring. So, as soon as the last snow melts, mix up a batch of this tonic. (This recipe makes enough for 2,500 square feet of lawn area. The lime and gypsum are available at garden/home centers and hardware stores.)

**50 lb. of pelletized lime**
**50 lb. of pelletized gypsum**
**5 lb. of Epsom salts**

Combine these ingredients, and apply the mixture using a hand-held broadcast spreader. Then wait at least two weeks before using any fertilizer.

## ● ROOT-PRUNING TONIC

After you root-prune any shrub, treat the wounds with this healing elixir.

**¼ lb. of Epsom salts**
**1 can of beer**
**4 tbsp. of instant tea granules**
**1 tbsp. of whiskey**
**1 tbsp. of baby shampoo**
**1 tbsp. of ammonia**
**1 tbsp. of hydrogen peroxide**
**2 gal. of very warm water**

Pour the Epsom salts evenly into the cuts, all the way around the plant. Then mix the remaining ingredients together in a bucket, and pour the solution over the Epsom salts.

## ● ROSE-ROUSING TONIC

After a bath in this potion, your bare-root roses will take off like gangbusters.

**1 vitamin $B_1$ tablet, dissolved in**
   **hot water**
**1 tbsp. of Epsom salts**
**1 tsp. of baby shampoo**
**1 gal. of water**

Mix all of these ingredients together in a bucket. Soak your roses' roots in the solution for at least 24 hours before you plant them.

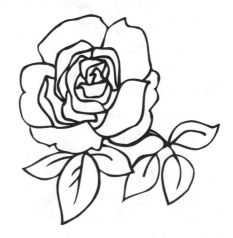

## ● ROSE-ROUSING TONIC II

When you can't wait a whole day to get your roses into the ground, use this instant formula.

**2 tbsp. of clear corn syrup**
**2 tsp. of dishwashing liquid**
**1 tsp. of ammonia**
**1 gal. of warm water**

Mix all of these ingredients in a bucket. Before planting your bare-root roses, soak them in the solution for about half an hour.

## ● ROSE START-UP TONIC

Here's the perfect meal to get your bushes off to a bright new beginning.

**½ gal. of warm tea**
**1 tbsp. of dishwashing liquid**
**1 tbsp. of hydrogen peroxide**
**1 tsp. of whiskey**
**1 tsp. of Vitamin B$_1$ Plant Starter**

Mix all of these ingredients together in a watering can, and pour the liquid all around the root zone of each newly planted (or transplanted) rose bush.

## ● ROSE TRANSPLANT TONIC

When you transplant roses, ease the transition to their new homes with this terrific tonic.

**½ can of beer**
**1 tbsp. of ammonia**
**1 tbsp. of instant tea granules**
**1 tbsp. of baby shampoo**
**1 gal. of water**

Mix all of these ingredients together, and add 1 cup of the solution to each hole at transplant time.

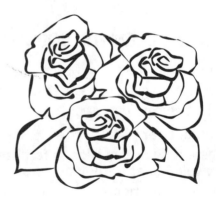

## ● ROT-PREVENTION TONIC

To fend off root rot all through your garden, add plenty of organic matter to the soil to ensure good drainage, and douse your plants' roots in early spring with this elixir.

**½ cup of antiseptic mouthwash**
**½ cup of baby shampoo**
**2 gal. of warm water**

Mix all of these ingredients in a watering can, and slowly pour the solution over each plant's root zone.

## ● ROYAL CLEMATIS COCKTAIL

Your clematis (a.k.a. the Queen of Climbers) will put on a regal show if you feed it this excellent elixir.

**1 can of beer**
**2 tbsp. of Fish Emulsion (a fertilizer available at garden centers)**
**4 tbsp. of ammonia**
**2 tbsp. of baby shampoo**

Mix all of these ingredients in a 2-gallon watering can, and fill the balance of the can with warm water. Pour the libation around the roots of your vine every three weeks or so throughout the growing season.

## ● RUST FUNGUS FIGHTER TONIC

Have your plants broken out in rust? After you've removed and destroyed the badly infected leaves, nix any lingering fungus with this formula.

**6 tbsp. of vegetable oil**
**2 tbsp. of baking soda**
**2 tbsp. of kelp extract**
**1 gal. of water**

Combine all of the ingredients, and pour the solution into a hand-held spray bottle. Spray the plants' foliage from top to bottom. Repeat every week to 10 days during damp or humid weather.

## ● SAFE-AND-SOUND PESTICIDE

Looking for a bad-bug killer that you *know* is harmless? Well, look no further! They don't come any safer than this. (That is, unless you're an aphid, spider mite, whitefly, or other pest!)

⅓ cup of cooking oil (any kind will do)
1 tsp. of baking soda
1 cup of water

Mix the oil and baking soda together. Then combine 2 teaspoons of this mixture with 1 cup of water in a hand-held spray bottle, and fire away when ready.

## ● SEED AND SOIL ENERGIZING TONIC

Once you've sown flower or vegetable seeds, indoors or out, give them an energy boost with this elixir.

1 tsp. of whiskey
1 tsp. of ammonia
1 tsp. of dishwashing liquid
1 qt. of weak tea

Mix all of these ingredients together, and pour the solution into a hand-held spray bottle. Shake it gently, and mist the surface of newly planted seed beds or plant containers.

## ● SEED SEND-OFF

When you start your seeds—indoors or out—give them this nourishing soak to start 'em out strong.

1 cup of white vinegar
1 tbsp. of baby shampoo or dishwashing liquid
2 cups of warm water

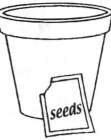

Mix the vinegar and baby shampoo or dishwashing liquid in the warm water. Soak your seeds in the solution overnight before planting them in well-prepared soil.

## ● SEED-STARTER TONIC

Flower and vegetable seeds germinate better and faster with this energizing pre-treatment.

1 tsp. of Epsom salts
1 tsp. of baby shampoo
1 qt. of weak tea

Combine all of the ingredients, and drop in your seeds. Put them in the refrigerator to soak for 24 hours before you plant them. Use a separate container for each kind of seed—that is, unless you want a casual mix, or you want to play "Name That Plant" when the seedlings come up!

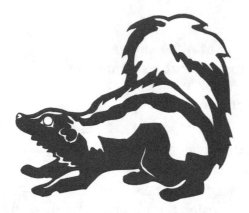

## ● SKUNK ODOR-OUT TONIC

When a skunk comes a-callin' and leaves some fragrant evidence behind, reach for this easy remedy.

**1 cup of bleach or vinegar**
**1 tbsp. of dishwashing liquid**
**2 ½ gal. of warm water**

Mix all of these ingredients in a bucket and thoroughly saturate walls, stairs, or anything else your local skunk has left his mark on.

**Caution:** Use this tonic only on nonliving things—not on pets or humans.

## ● SLUGWEISER

Beer is a classic bait for slug and snail traps, but what attracts the slimy marauders isn't the thought of a good time at the local pub—it's the sugar and yeast in the brew. So, don't raid the fridge to fill your traps. Use this libation instead.

**1 lb. of brown sugar**
**½ package (1 ½ tsp.) of dry yeast**
**Warm water**

Pour the sugar and yeast into a 1-gallon container, fill it with warm water, and let it sit for two days, uncovered. Sink some shallow cans into the ground up to their rims, pour in the brew, and watch the culprits belly up to the bar!

## ● SPRING SHRUB TONIC

When winter has finally passed, help your shrubs spring into action by watering them with the following elixir.

**4 tbsp. of bourbon or other whiskey**
**4 tbsp. of instant tea granules**
**2 tbsp. of dishwashing liquid**
**2 gal. of warm water**

Mix all of these ingredients in a watering can, and pour the solution slowly onto the root zone of each shrub. (This recipe makes enough tonic to feed one shrub.)

## ● SPRING SOIL ENERGIZER TONIC

Before you plant your vegetable garden, give the soil a drink of this potent potion.

**1 can of beer**
**½ cup of regular cola (not diet)**
**½ cup of dishwashing liquid**
**½ cup of antiseptic mouthwash**
**¼ tsp. of instant tea granules**

Mix all of these ingredients in your 20 gallon hose-end sprayer, and saturate the soil. Wait two weeks before you start planting. (This recipe makes enough to cover 100 square feet of garden area.)

## ● STRAWBERRY SHORTCUT TONIC

This terrific tonic is a shortcut to a bumper strawberry harvest.

**1 can of beer**
**¼ cup of cold coffee**
**2 tbsp. of dishwashing liquid**
**2 gal. of water**

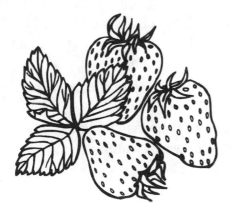

Mix all of the ingredients together in a bucket, and soak the berries' bare roots in the solution for about 10 minutes before you plant them. After you've tucked them into their holes, dribble the leftover solution on the soil around them.

## ● SUPER SLUG SPRAY

Slugs driving you crazy? Pull out this heavy artillery.

**½ cup of ammonia**
**1 tbsp. of Murphy's Oil Soap®**
**1½ cups of water**

Pour all of the ingredients into a hand-held spray bottle, and shake well. Then take aim, and fire!

## ● SUPER SPIDER-MITE MIX

When tiny spider mites are causing big mischief in your garden, reach for this recipe.

**4 cups of wheat flour**
**½ cup of buttermilk**
**5 gal. of water**

Mix all of these ingredients together, pour the mixture into a hand-held spray bottle, and mist-spray your plants to the point of run-off.

## ● TIMELY TOMATO TONIC

This powerful powder will help your tomato plants fend off nasty diseases.

**3 cups of compost**
**½ cup of Epsom salts**
**1 tbsp. of baking soda**
**½ cup of powdered nonfat milk**

Combine the first three ingredients in a bucket, and add a handful of the mix to the planting hole. After planting, sprinkle a little of the powdered milk on top of the soil. Repeat every few weeks during the growing season.

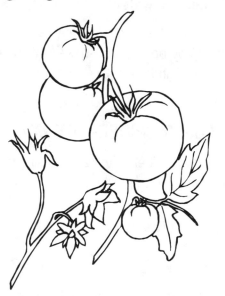

## ● TRANSPLANT TONIC

For a tree or shrub, being transplanted is a shocking experience. This soothing drink will ease the stress of going from a nursery pot, or the bare-root wrappings, to the wide-open spaces of your yard or garden.

**⅓ cup of hydrogen peroxide**
**¼ cup of bourbon or other whiskey**
**¼ cup of instant tea granules**
**¼ cup of baby shampoo**
**2 tbsp. of Fish Emulsion (a fertilizer available at garden centers)**
**1 gal. of water**

Mix all of these ingredients in a bucket, and pour the solution into the new planting hole.

## ● TREE WOUND STERILIZER TONIC

Any time you cut diseased tissue from a tree or shrub, kill lingering germs with this powerful potion.

**¼ cup of antiseptic mouthwash**
**¼ cup of ammonia**
**¼ cup of dishwashing liquid**
**1 gal. of warm water**

Mix all of the ingredients, pour the solution into a hand-held spray bottle, and drench the places where you've pruned off limbs or branches.

## ● VEGETABLE GARDEN BEDTIME TONIC

When you put your vegetable garden to bed for the winter, top it with a thick layer of organic mulch, then give it this nightcap.

**1 can of regular cola (not diet)**
**1 cup of dishwashing liquid**
**¼ cup of ammonia**

Mix all of these ingredients in your 20 gallon hose-end sprayer, and fill the balance of the jar with warm water. Then spray until the mulch is saturated.

## ● WILD WEED WIPEOUT

Here's the perfect recipe for nixing those *really* stubborn weeds.

**2 tbsp. of gin**
**2 tbsp. of vinegar**
**2 tbsp. of dishwashing liquid**
**1 qt. of hot water**

Mix all of these ingredients together, pour the solution into a hand-held spray bottle, and blast those weeds to you-know-where!

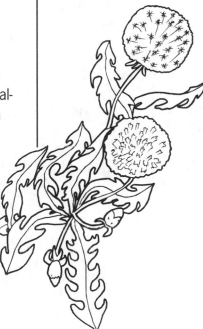

# INDEX

## A

# D

# I

# R

## T